PATHOGENIC POLICING

MEDICAL ANTHROPOLOGY: HEALTH, INEQUALITY, AND SOCIAL JUSTICE

Series editor: Lenore Manderson

Books in the Medical Anthropology series are concerned with social patterns of and social responses to ill health, disease, and suffering, and how social exclusion and social justice shape health and healing outcomes. The series is designed to reflect the diversity of contemporary medical anthropological research and writing, and will offer scholars a forum to publish work that showcases the theoretical sophistication, methodological soundness, and ethnographic richness of the field.

Books in the series may include studies on the organization and movement of peoples, technologies, and treatments, how inequalities pattern access to these, and how individuals, communities and states respond to various assaults on wellbeing, including from illness, disaster, and violence.

Ellen Block and Will McGrath, *Infected Kin: Orphan Care and AIDS in Lesotho*
Jessica Hardin, *Faith and the Pursuit of Health: Cardiometabolic Disorders in Samoa*
Carina Heckert, *Fault Lines of Care: Gender, HIV, and Global Health in Bolivia*
Alison Heller, *Fistula Politics: Birthing Injuries and the Quest for Continence in Niger*
Nolan Kline, *Pathogenic Policing: Immigration Enforcement and Health in the U.S. South*
Joel Christian Reed, *Landscapes of Activism: Civil Society and HIV and AIDS Care in Northern Mozambique*
Beatriz M. Reyes-Foster, *Psychiatric Encounters: Madness and Modernity in Yucatan, Mexico*
Sonja van Wichelen, *Legitimating Life: Adoption in the Age of Globalization and Biotechnology*
Lesley Jo Weaver, *Sugar and Tension: Diabetes and Gender in Modern India*
Andrea Whittaker, *International Surrogacy as Disruptive Industry in Southeast Asia*

PATHOGENIC POLICING

Immigration Enforcement and Health in the U.S. South

NOLAN KLINE

RUTGERS UNIVERSITY PRESS

New Brunswick, Camden, and Newark, New Jersey, and London

Library of Congress Cataloging-in-Publication Data

Names: Kline, Nolan, 1986– author.
Title: Pathogenic policing : immigration enforcement and health in the US
    South / Nolan Kline.
Other titles: Medical anthropology (New Brunswick, N.J.)
Description: New Brunswick, New Jersey : Rutgers University Press, [2019] |
    Series: Medical anthropology | Includes bibliographical references and
    index.
Identifiers: LCCN 2018047933| ISBN 9780813595337 (hardcover : alk. paper) |
    ISBN 9780813595320 (pbk. : alk. paper)
Subjects: | MESH: Health Policy | Public Policy | Undocumented Immigrants |
    Emigration and Immigration—legislation & jurisprudence | Healthcare
    Disparities | Health Services Accessibility | Law Enforcement | Georgia
Classification: LCC RA448.5.I44 | NLM WA 540 AG4 | DDC 362.1086/912—dc23
LC record available at https://catalog.loc.gov/vwebv/search?searchCode=LCCN&
searchArg=2018047933&searchType=1&permalink=y

A British Cataloging-in-Publication record for this book is available from
the British Library.

www.rutgersuniversitypress.org

Manufactured in the United States of America

For the GLAHRiadores

CONTENTS

FOREWORD

LENORE MANDERSON

Medical Anthropology: Health, Inequality, and Social Justice is a new series from Rutgers University Press, designed to capture the diversity of contemporary medical anthropological research and writing. The beauty of ethnography is its capacity, through storytelling, to make sense of suffering as a social experience and to set it in context. Central to our focus in this series on health and illness, inequality, and social justice, therefore, is the way in which social structures and ideologies shape the likelihood and impact of infections, injuries, bodily ruptures and disease, chronic conditions and disability, treatment and care, social repair and death.

The brief for this series is broad. The books are concerned with health and illness, healing practices, and access to care, but the authors illustrate too the importance of context—of geography, physical condition, service availability, and income. Health and illness are social facts; the circumstances of the maintenance and loss of health are always and everywhere shaped by structural, global, and local relations. Society, culture, economy, and political organization as much as ecology shape the variance of illness, disability, and disadvantage. But as medical anthropologists have long illustrated, the relationships of social context and health status are complex. In addressing these questions, the authors in this series showcase the theoretical sophistication, methodological rigor, and empirical richness of the field while expanding a map of illness and social and institutional life to illustrate the effects of material conditions and social meanings in troubling and surprising ways.

The books in the series move across social circumstances, health conditions, and geography, and their intersections and interactions, to demonstrate how individuals, communities, and states manage assaults on wellbeing. The books reflect medical anthropology as a constantly changing field of scholarship, drawing on research diversely in residential and virtual communities, in clinics and laboratories, and in emergency care and public health settings, with service providers, individual healers, and households, with social bodies, human bodies, and biologies. While medical anthropology once concentrated on systems of healing, particular diseases, and embodied experiences, today the field has expanded to include environmental disaster and war, science, technology and faith, gender-based violence, and forced migration. Curiosity about the body and its vicissitudes remains a pivot for our work, but our concerns are with the location of bodies in social life and how social structures, temporal imperatives, and shifting exigencies shape life courses. This dynamic field reflects an ethics of the discipline to address these pressing issues of our time.

Globalization has contributed to the complexity of influences on health outcomes; it (re)produces social and economic relations that institutionalize poverty, unequal conditions of everyday life and work, and environments in which diseases increase or subside. Globalization patterns the movement and relations of peoples, technologies and knowledge, and programs and treatments; it shapes differences in health experience and outcomes across space; it informs and amplifies inequalities at individual and country levels. Global forces and local inequalities compound and constantly load on individuals to impact on their physical and mental health, and on their households and communities. At the same time, as the subtitle of this series indicates, we are concerned with questions of social exclusion and inclusion, social justice and repair, again both globally and in local settings. The books will challenge readers to reflect not only on sickness and suffering, deficit and despair, but also on resistance and restitution—on how people respond to injustices and evade the fault lines that might seem to predetermine life outcomes. While not all of the books take this direction, the aim is to widen the frame within which we conceptualize embodiment and suffering.

As this book goes to press, globally almost 70 million people are classified as refugees or asylum seekers. Most are displaced from their homes within their countries of birth and intraregionally. An estimated 10 million people are stateless, not all included in this prior group; one-third of these are children, born in countries where their births cannot be registered. Many of these people are residing in the global north, in countries that might seem to offer them safety, security, and care.

Untold numbers of people fall outside of such classifications as refugee or asylum seeker. They are resident in countries without government permission to do so, sometimes having overstayed visas as workers or students, other times having entered the country without complying with national border policies and local laws. The bundling of such people as "illegal immigrants"—even as irregular, undocumented, or unauthorized immigrants—disguises the circumstances that lead to their migration, the precarity of their journeys, and the conditions in which they live on resettlement. In *Pathogenic Policing: Immigration Enforcement and Health in the U.S. South*, Nolan Kline turns to the rule of law, and shows how those without legal documents are exposed to a wide range of restrictions, deprivations, risks and vulnerabilities. For economic reasons and because of their vulnerable civil status, undocumented immigrants often live precariously in substandard housing on the periphery of cities, where transport and services are especially poor. They work in dangerous conditions, underpaid and without contracts. They are subject to discrimination and marginalization. They are typically denied access to health care, social services, justice and education, since even with the right theoretically to access such services, to do so exposes them to possible detention and deportation. The constant surveillance to which immigrants are subject is a key factor in preventing them from seeking support, including health care. Family groups and everyday relationships are routinely ruptured as some individuals are apprehended and returned to their countries of origin; others are left behind. Fear of arrest, detention, deportation, and family separation shapes their everyday lives.

In *Pathogenic Policing: Immigration Enforcement and Health in the U.S. South*, Nolan Kline illustrates how, in the state of Georgia, a simple document—a driver's license—stands as evidence of the right to services. The absence of a license is, conversely, prima facie evidence of a person's "illegal" status, from which he or she is subject to police protocol and processes, with deportation the usual and expected outcome. But having or not having a driver's license can be proved only on request, once a person is intercepted while driving a car. People who "look" like an immigrant and so assumed to be "illegal" are routinely stopped by police, and so undocumented immigrants avoid the law by avoiding driving, so limiting where and if they work, when and how they shop, and whether they seek health care for themselves or others in their family. Immigration enforcement policy therefore shapes immigrants' health and interpersonal relationships, forcing them to survive by stealth, with impacts not only on the lives of individual immigrants but also on health providers, immigrant rights groups, health insurance and related programs, and clinics and hospitals. In *Pathogenic Policing* Nolan Kline reminds us of the multiple ways by which people are deprived of their health as a human right.

PATHOGENIC POLICING

INTRODUCTION
"They Will Stop You"

At a weekly meeting of the Georgia Latino Alliance for Human Rights (GLAHR), Adelina,[1] the executive director, reminded everyone of how important it was to drive carefully. She had just taken a phone call on the GLAHR hotline in which a woman named Esme asked for help regarding her husband, Alvaro. A local police officer had stopped Alvaro for having a broken taillight. Esme swore she had checked the taillight and that it had been working perfectly the week before the officer pulled over her husband. As in any routine traffic stop, the officer asked Alvaro for his driver's license. But Alvaro is undocumented, and since Georgia does not allow undocumented immigrants to obtain driver's licenses, he was unable to produce the requested identification. The officer arrested Alvaro for driving without a license, and when Esme called GLAHR, he was being held in a county jail. Esme feared Alvaro would be deported to Mexico, and she asked Adelina for help figuring out what would happen to him. Adelina informed her that the U.S. Immigration and Customs Enforcement (ICE) had forty-eight hours to put a detainer on Alvaro, and she gave Esme the phone number of a lawyer to consult. Shortly after hanging up the phone, Adelina walked out of her office and went to the room full of GLAHR members—collectively known as GLAHRiadores, a linguistic play on "gladiators" (or *gladiadores* in Spanish)—where she discussed Esme's situation.

"*Compañeros* [friends], we all know how important it is to drive carefully, *sí?*" Adelina asked, sparking a conversation on a frequently discussed topic. She and other GLAHRiadores reiterated strategies for avoiding police scrutiny, such as ensuring tail and brake lights worked, using turn signals, driving under the speed limit, and always wearing seatbelts. "*Sí, es muy importante* [yes, it is very important]. You have to make sure everything is functioning properly on your car, always wear a seatbelt, and drive under the speed limit. They [the police] will stop you."

The conversation at GLAHR that night summarized what many immigrants in Atlanta identified as a problem threatening their communities: aggressive policing tactics that demanded political and social action. For the GLAHRiadores, aggressive police practices include more than just stopping immigrants for actions many people in the United States do routinely, like driving over the speed limit, not using a turn signal, and not coming to a complete stop at a stop sign. They also include police setting up *retenes* (checkpoints) outside Latinx (a gender-neutral form of Latino/a) neighborhoods, churches, apartment complexes, trailer parks, and shopping centers to stop every driver who looked Latinx.[2] More broadly, policing fits into a context of anti-immigrant sentiment that has become codified in state laws and federal statutes. These policies, representing an overall anti-immigrant response to people like Adelina, Esme, and the GLAHRiadores, operate locally through police actions and have sweeping consequences for immigrants, their families, and health facilities across Georgia.

In this book, I examine the multiple impacts of immigrant policing in Atlanta—the metropolitan heart of the U.S. South. Immigrant policing comprises policies and police practices that render undocumented immigrants visible to authorities for arrest and potential deportation (Kline 2017). These activities ultimately shape undocumented immigrants' wellbeing and have numerous health-related consequences that reverberate throughout the communities in which they live, and affect institutions that all populations rely on, like hospitals. In examining the numerous health-related impacts of immigrant policing, I consider immigrant policing as a form of health policy and trace its consequences through multiple settings. As medical anthropologists Arachu Castro and Merrill Singer note (2004), policy is a set of "guidelines implemented by a social institution intended to set a direction for action," and health policy can include "policy with another purpose but nonetheless having a direct impact on health" (xi). As I show in this book, immigration enforcement efforts are health policies since they have several health-related impacts and the consequences of immigrant policing extend beyond undocumented immigrants, especially in the largest city in the Deep South[3], which is home to an aggressive immigrant policing regime.

The immigration enforcement regime I describe in Atlanta reflects an overall hostile immigration context in the United States, especially under President Donald Trump. Trump's approach to immigration has often reaffirmed racialized notions of difference and supported race-based police practices. For example, in 2017, Trump pardoned Arizona former sheriff Joe Arpaio for his conviction for criminal contempt. Arpaio, famous for racially profiling Latinx drivers and operating his county jail under abusive conditions, had been convicted of defying a court order to cease detaining people based on suspicion of their immigration status (Pérez-Peña 2017). In pardoning Arpaio, Trump vindicated the former sheriff's racial profiling practices that some law enforcement agencies in the Atlanta area modeled.

LAYERED IMMIGRANT POLICING IN ATLANTA

Atlanta is a relatively new destination for Latinx immigrants and is home to layered immigration enforcement efforts comprising state laws and federal programs that operate locally. As the ninth-largest metropolitan area in the United States, with the nation's tenth-largest economy and one of the top fifty economies in the world (Bureau of Economic Analysis 2016; Chapman 2014), Atlanta is a booming metropolis in an otherwise largely rural state (Georgia State Office of Rural Health, n.d.). It is also the capital of Georgia, where immigration enforcement laws were drafted and passed in a gold-domed statehouse outside of which GLAHRiadores protested, held marches, and demanded change to state and federal immigration laws.

As I describe in the next chapter, the United States features a large federal government with individual states having their own sovereignty, but some policy issues are typically the exclusive domain of the federal government. In the United States, immigration concerns have historically been a matter reserved for federal oversight, but in recent years, immigration enforcement laws have become more commonly passed in state legislatures (Lopes and Thomas 2014), including in Georgia. Layered immigration enforcement laws at state and federal levels have created multiple threats of discovery for undocumented immigrants: "multiple *migras*"—a way to refer to immigration enforcement in Spanish—or a "poli-migra," as the sociologist Cecilia Menjívar has described (2014, 5). The current "poli-migra" operating in several U. S. states is an amalgam of federal statutes, state laws, local ordinances, and police activities targeting undocumented immigrants. It intensifies immigration enforcement and enhances immigrants' likelihood of encountering enforcement agents (Menjívar 2014, 5). More than just ramping up policing efforts to catch undocumented immigrants, layered immigration enforcement efforts allow police officers to become immigration authorities, amplifying the effects of metaphorically moving the U.S.-Mexico border and its risks of apprehension inwardly and locally (Leerkes, Leach, and Bachmeier 2012; Coleman 2007). Deputizing police officers results in eroded trust between law enforcement agents and some immigrant communities, and in Atlanta, some immigrants would not call police if they were robbed, assaulted, or otherwise victimized because they associated police with the potential for deportation.

Layered immigration enforcement regimes ultimately influence undocumented immigrants' social disadvantages that impact their long- and short-term opportunities (Menjívar 2014), including access to health services and their overall wellbeing (Cleaveland and Ihara 2012; Berk et al. 2000). In Atlanta, layered immigrant policing efforts not only altered some undocumented immigrants' health behaviors and interpersonal relationships but further implicated health providers in policing efforts and impacted the entire medical safety net that serves all Atlanta-area residents.

Although some state immigration laws have increased immigrants' access to social services such as driver's licenses and in-state tuition for undocumented college students (Marrow 2012; Abrego 2008), others have focused on legislating exclusions (Menjívar 2014; Walker and Leitner 2011). In southern states like Georgia, which serve as new destinations for immigrants (Leerkes, Leach, and Bachmeier 2012), legislation has tended to be exclusion focused. Georgia has passed several state laws limiting undocumented immigrants' access to social services and followed other states, such as Arizona, in passing legislation that effectively permitted racial profiling of Latinx immigrants. When Arizona's notorious Senate Bill (SB) 1070 passed in 2010, it was one of the most publicized state laws in the United States and was touted as the "toughest immigration law in the country" (Campbell 2011, 1). SB 1070 made it a crime for an immigrant to be present without carrying required documentation and mandated that law enforcement officers assess a person's immigration status if they suspected the individual of being undocumented. These two provisions earned the Arizona legislation the nickname of the "papers, please" law (see, for example, Warmerdam 2016), a reference to Nazi-era scrutiny of citizens in everyday spaces. The year after Arizona passed SB 1070, Georgia passed a similar law, House Bill (HB) 87, which also granted local law officers the authority to assess a person's immigration status.

Georgia's immigration laws like HB 87 respond to a fast-growing immigrant population compared with those of other states. As I describe in the next chapter, the Latinx population in Georgia has more than doubled since the year 2000, reaching 853,689 in 2010, and with approximately sixty-four percent (547,400) living in metropolitan Atlanta (U.S. Census Bureau 2010).[4] Although Latinx immigration to the state has been associated with agricultural work since the 1940s (Walcott and Murphy 2006), immigration to the Atlanta area rose during the 1970s and 1980s fueled by the poultry, textile, and construction industries (Yarbrough 2010). Throughout the 1990s, Atlanta experienced significant economic growth driven by the construction, finance, transportation, and utility industries (Odem 2008), and Latinx immigration continued to increase, especially from Mexico, where an oil-related economic boom ended (Walcott and Murphy 2006). As the Latinx population in Atlanta grew, so did African and Asian immigrant populations, and Atlanta became home to the largest immigrant population and largest Latinx community in the U.S. South (Yarbrough 2010).[5]

The number of Mexican immigrants arriving in Atlanta in the 1990s was also partly due to a need for construction laborers to ensure a timely beginning of the 1996 Summer Olympic Games (Wickert 2016; Olsson 2014; Associated Press 2010; Grillo 2010; Bess and Shelton 2008). Before the opening of the Olympics, city and state officials encountered a labor shortage and feared construction projects would not be completed on time. Concerned about international embarrassment, Georgia officials met with Mexican governmental representatives and requested an intervention. As Teodoro Maus, the former consul of Mexico and more frequently called *Don* (a term of endearment) Teo by those who know him, explained to me: "They asked us to get workers from Mexico to come and help with construction. They were behind schedule and nothing was going to be completed in time, so they said 'just get us workers and we'll sort out the immigration stuff later.'" The promise to "sort out the immigration stuff later" was an empty one, as Don Teo later learned. "We agreed to spread the word," he explained, "and all over Mexico you started seeing billboards pop up that said 'Georgia is hiring,' and things like that. And of course, they never fixed the immigration stuff, like they said they would."

As Don Teo suggested, the construction sector provided a large number of jobs for Atlanta's Latinx population; in 2000, Latinxs accounted for approximately forty-five percent of the construction workforce in the area's counties (Odem 2008). Upon completing Olympics-related projects, Latinx immigrants continued to work in construction and participated in Atlanta's housing boom. The economic downturn of the 2000s, however, included the housing market crash and concomitant decline in construction projects. The national economic crisis and construction halt in Atlanta fueled anti-immigrant sentiment in the metropolitan area. Policy makers I interviewed for this book largely explained the economic downturn as the impetus for a deluge of anti-immigrant laws, which has included fifteen separate pieces of legislation between 2006 and 2017 (Project South, n.d.), the most notorious of which is HB 87.

In 2011, Georgia governor Nathan Deal fulfilled a campaign promise of enacting an "Arizona-style" immigration law by signing the Illegal Immigration Reform and Enforcement Act of 2011, more commonly referred to as HB 87.[6] Building on previous Georgia laws and duplicating key features of Arizona's SB 1070, HB 87 requires immigrants to carry proof of legal status at all times and compels police officers to stop anyone suspected of being undocumented. The law requires private employers receiving public funds to verify employees' legal status, and allows the public to sue state officials who do not enforce laws related to immigration matters (Browne and Odem 2012). It also created the Immigration Enforcement and Review Board (IERB), a committee to ensure compliance with the law and hear public complaints, whose public meetings I attended while doing the research for this book. HB 87 also criminalized any assistance to undocumented immigrants, potentially implicating taxi drivers, charitable organization leaders, and others who provide types of aid or services. The provisions surrounding assistance and transportation prohibited health care professionals from providing any type of publicly financed, nonemergency health service, effectively criminalizing some health care providers' professional actions and extending efforts to control undocumented immigrants into medical realms by making medical personnel agents of documentation status surveillance.[7]

In addition to HB 87 and other immigration enforcement laws, the Georgia legislature proposed banning undocumented youth participating in the Deferred

Action for Childhood Arrivals (DACA) program from obtaining driver's licenses (Foley 2014), and the Georgia Board of Regents banned undocumented students from attending Georgia's most selective universities, including the University of Georgia (Brown 2010). Georgia legislators also proposed laws (SB 160 and HB 125) that threatened undocumented immigrants' abilities to open bank accounts, rent apartments, or turn on utilities, as I describe in chapter 2. The state has banned so-called sanctuary cities, or cities that attempt to limit municipal employees' interactions with immigration enforcement officials, and passed a law to demand local governments cooperate with federal immigration officials in order to receive state funding. In short, Georgia policy makers have made a concerted effort to signal to undocumented immigrants that they are not welcome in the Peach State.

State laws and education policies, however, are only one portion of the multi-layered immigrant policing regime operating in Georgia. Adding to Georgia's state laws are federal immigration statutes and programs that operate on local levels: section 287(g) of the Immigration and Nationality Act, and Secure Communities. Section 287(g) allows for state and local law enforcement agencies to act as immigration enforcement officers through agreements with the Department of Homeland Security and the ICE (Shahshahani 2009).[8] As I describe in greater detail in the next chapter, 287(g)-agreements allow for simple arrests, such as traffic violations like the one Alvaro allegedly committed, to become potential triggers for deportation. Similarly, Secure Communities allows for simple arrests to turn into deportations by sending arrestees' fingerprints that are taken in local jails to federal immigration authorities. Federal officials then use the fingerprints they receive to assess an arrestee's immigration status. In Georgia, six counties participate in the 287(g) program (Bartow, Cobb, Floyd, Gwinnett, Hall, and Whitfield), five of which are in the Atlanta metropolitan area, and all jurisdictions in the United States currently participate in the Secure Communities program.[9] The effects of both programs are a localized immigration enforcement regime that makes the threat of deportation associated with elements of daily life, like driving to work, a grocery store, place of worship, school, or home, as demonstrated by what happened to Alvaro, and the reports of *retenes* that occur in Latinx neighborhoods (Stuesse and Coleman 2014).

POLICY, POWER, AND POPULATION CONTROL

The multiple and overlapping immigrant policing measures in Atlanta speak to national anxieties over immigration that converge with broader topics related to race, health, economics, and other social phenomena. The proliferation of legislation targeting immigrants, and the numerous immigrant-policing techniques designed to control immigrant populations demand attention to better understand how these efforts affect undocumented immigrants and institutions such as health care organizations, and may have hidden consequences. In this book, I argue that immigration enforcement policy creates an intentional fear response in undocumented immigrants that shapes their health, and the health-related impacts of immigrant policing extend beyond immigrants to affect immigrants' interpersonal relationships, health providers' professional practice, nongovernment organizations (NGOs), hospitals, and the overall health system. By focusing on immigrant policing and its numerous consequences, I show how, as immigration scholar Nicholas De Genova asserts, "illegality" itself is a sociopolitical condition (2002, 423), and I further demonstrate how policies that produce illegality and exploit immigrants' fears of deportation have numerous consequences that are not confined to people with undocumented status. In other words, the vulnerabilities and instability of illegality can extend beyond undocumented immigrants and affect several populations and social institutions. To advance this argument, I borrow from theories of biopolitics and citizenship.

Biopolitics, as philosopher Michel Foucault writes, refers to the ways in which populations are divided and categorized for efficient means of control. The term refers to how power can be applied over groups of people and their bodies as a collective, rather than as individuals (Foucault 2003). Foucault considers how power works to categorize groups of people by using socially and culturally constructed ideas like race and sexual orientation (2003, 242). Biopolitics, then, can be understood as an application of power over a population, or what Foucault calls "biopower" (1978, 140). Immigrant policing efforts, which hinge on notions of difference based on documentation status and race, are a form of biopower that attempt to govern or control immigrants. Immigrant policing specifically attempts to govern immigrants through fear, aiming to make them afraid of living their daily lives and seeking health services when needed.

As Foucault argues, categories like race allow for human populations to be divided for more efficient control and for determining which population receives investment and which does not. This type of power over the population, or biopolitics, ultimately allows for determining who can metaphorically live and die, and Foucault referred to this antagonism as "race-war logic," a logic that at the most basic level asserts that in order for one group to be successful, another must not be. In the case of undocumented immigrants in the United States, whose immigration status is often conflated with a form of racial otherness and assumed associations with Mexico, Central America, or South America, harsh immigrant policing regimes are a way of symbolically investing in the lives of white nonimmigrants while simultaneously divesting from the lives of nonwhite undocumented immigrants.

In addition to being a way of governing populations, immigrant policing also serves as a way to establish a type of relationship between undocumented immigrants and governmental authorities. This relationship can be understood through the analytical frame of citizenship. Though commonly understood as a synonym for national identity, for social scientists, citizenship refers to a relationship between a person or population and a polity, encompassing sets of rights and entitlements, and including notions of belonging to a specific group (Isin and Turner 2002). Immigrant policing efforts, which make undocumented immigrants fearful of using health services, attempt to fashion immigrants into citizens who hesitate to make demands for services. This form of citizenship ultimately comports with the basics of neoliberalism: the economic ideology characterized by shrinking governmental services and championing notions of individual responsibility (Harvey 2007; Hyatt 2001; Wacquant 2001; Maskovsky 2000; Schneider 1999). In governing immigrants through fear, immigrant policing efforts aim to produce a neoliberal citizen—a citizen who will refuse to make demands on governmental agencies for publicly funded health services and instead find alternate, personally funded forms of services like health care (also see Inda and Dowling 2013, 4). Producing a neoliberal citizen has sweeping consequences that extend beyond individuals to affect relationships, health providers, and health care institutions.

MEDICAL ANTHROPOLOGY, PUBLIC HEALTH, AND ENGAGED ETHNOGRAPHY

As a medical anthropologist with a public health training, I started the research that resulted in this book curious to know how immigrant policing itself might be a health determinant like other social phenomena. I suspected that immigrant policing, like other social determinants of health, impacted more people and institutions than individual immigrants, and I sought a methodological framework that could consider the multiple pathways of immigration enforcement. Both anthropology and public health offer frameworks for tracing an idea or problem through multiple spaces. For example, anthropologists use multi-sited ethnography to not just deeply examine one site but instead broaden a traditional field site to multiple geographic and social spaces (Marcus 1995). Similarly, anthropologists who study policy do so by examining how policy and associated political interests move "through" multiple spaces (Wedel et al. 2005). For my fieldwork, I borrowed from multi-sited ethnography and the anthropology of policy to trace the numerous impacts of immigrant policing across multiple social spaces, going to immigrants' homes, community organizations, hospitals, and the state capital. Similarly, leveraging my public health background, I used a health sciences model that conceptualizes how to conduct research at different social levels, borrowing from the social ecological model of health (see, for example, McLeroy et al. 1988), to consider the numerous individual, interpersonal, organizational, community, and policy-related impacts of immigrant policing. Combined, the multi-sited ethnography and social ecological model of health perspectives led me to talk to policy makers, health providers, immigrant rights organization leaders, undocumented immigrants, and other groups of people who could all speak to the numerous impacts of immigrant policing. By merging these perspectives,

I was able to methodically map out individuals and institutions for ethnographic inquiry and similarly add ethnographic richness to a health sciences model used to understand how health is situated within numerous social contexts.

Altogether, during the year of fieldwork between 2012 and 2013, I conducted over 115 interviews with health providers, Latinx immigrants, staff at NGOs, hospital staff, state agency workers, state legislators, immigrant rights allies, business owners impacted by *retenes*, and taxi drivers who witnessed firsthand the consequences of making roadways and other everyday spaces possible sites of deportation.[10] I also engaged in hundreds of hours of participant observation, which entailed attending weekly meetings of local immigrant rights groups; speaking with lobbyists and attending events inside the Georgia state capital; attending meetings with clinicians, public health officials, and community health advocates in health facilities; attending political demonstrations; volunteering with local activist groups; and participating in other activities that further shaped my understanding of immigrant policing. In addition to interviews and participant observation experiences, I conducted a media analysis of major news stories related to immigration policies.[11] Combined, the research that resulted in this book developed my overall understanding of the multiple health-related impacts of immigrant policing.

In tracing the impacts of immigrant policing, I further adopted a perspective of engaged and activist anthropology. Engaged and activist approaches to anthropological research erase notions of anthropologists as neutral participant observers (Sanford and Angel-Ajani 2006; Scheper-Hughes 2004) and instead build relationships of accountability and reciprocity between anthropologists and informants (Pulido 2008). Among the basic expectations of engaged scholarship are a researcher's meaningful contribution to participants, inclusion of participants in each phase of the research, and critical reflection of self and of the research (Hale 2008). This perspective arises out of a stance that generating knowledge alone cannot effect social change (Gordon 1991), and as a result, researchers are inserted into relationships with expectations (Pulido 2008). Those expectations can entail sharing a common political goal, typically one that confronts and attempts to eliminate inequalities produced through divisions based on race, class, sex, sexual orientation, and gender (Hale 2008). In the research that resulted in this book, the common political goal I shared with members and leaders of immigrant rights organizations was to end legislation and police practices that interfere with undocumented immigrants' daily lives, and more broadly, to end the systematic discrimination of undocumented Latinx and other immigrant groups in the United States.

Engaged and activist approaches are especially consonant with medical anthropological work. Critical medical anthropologists in particular have a long history of situating health within a political context in order to change "culturally inappropriate, oppressive and exploitative patterns in the health arena and beyond"

(Singer 1995, 81). Drawing from my training as a medical anthropologist, I embraced engaged and activist anthropology methodologies, and I was inspired by multi-sited techniques to trace the multiple pathways of immigrant policing. To do so, I joined immigrant rights and health activist organizations in the Atlanta area and participated in their major events, got to know their members, and shared their political causes. I worked most closely with GLAHR, whose leaders and members shared their experiences with me and welcomed me as a researcher, volunteer, and activist. I also worked closely with members of the Georgia Immigrant and Refugee Rights Coalition (GIRRC), which was active from 2009 to 2013, and coordinated communication among a number of organizations expressing a commitment to advancing immigrant rights. Through GLAHR and GIRRC, I met leaders of health-related organizations and activist groups who were willing to share their insights with me about the consequences of immigrant policing. These organizations included the Hispanic Health Coalition of Georgia, the only state-wide organization to focus on Latinx health; Caminar Latino, a family and intimate partner violence organization; the Partnership Against Domestic Violence; the Clinic for Education, Treatment, and Prevention of Addiction (CETPA), a mental health services and addiction prevention organization; and Cobb United for Change Coalition (CUCC), an organization dedicated to improving the lives of Cobb County residents.[12]

My involvement with these organizations connected me to a larger activist network in Atlanta that has a deep and rich history. Atlanta was a major hub for activist organizing during the U.S. civil rights movement and was home to prominent civil rights leaders, most notably Martin Luther King, Jr. As I became more involved with GLAHR and attended various immigrant rights events, I began recognizing people from organizations across Atlanta. One CUCC member explained, "Everyone knows everyone, and it's the same group of people at all the meetings!" My connection to GLAHR, GIRRC, and other groups resulted in me getting invitations to attend events that were not necessarily directly related to immigration but were within the scope of my political ideals and were activities other Atlanta-area activists thought were important for me to experience. This included, for example, attending a service at the historic Ebenezer Baptist Church to hear a sermon about ending police violence against black men and women. Invitations like this demonstrated how the activist civil society network in Atlanta sometimes operated: people from various organizations dedicated to specific causes, like racial justice or immigrant rights, would support other organizations' efforts in different capacities, including attending specific events.

Not all of the organizations I became familiar with are represented equally in this book, and of them all, I worked most closely with GLAHR. Adelina and Don Teo founded GLAHR in 1999, after the two of them met when Don Teo was looking for leaders to engage in advocacy for Georgia's Latinx community. "The first thing we did was deliver a petition to Governor Roy Barnes to get driver's licenses for undocumented immigrants," Adelina recalled, telling me about GLAHR's history. "I drove around the state, going door to door and got more than 30,000 people to sign. That's how I got to know the community, and when I realized that outside of Atlanta, the Latinx community didn't know what was going on in Georgia." Aiming to spread information to Latinx immigrants across Georgia and to begin community-organizing efforts, Adelina and Don Teo formed GLAHR and immediately began putting together political marches and rallies, including a 2001 march in the Atlanta suburb of Doraville, where they petitioned for immigrants to receive driver's licenses. Adelina and Don Teo continued to organize political events, and Adelina routinely made trips across the state to visit communities outside Atlanta.

As part of GLAHR's work, Adelina helps develop *comités populares*: local organizing groups focused on education, leadership training, and consciousness raising. Through my participation in GLAHR, I assisted Adelina and GLAHRiadores in organizing and attending political marches, contributed to a community-based art installation themed around undocumented immigrants' rights and experiences, wrote grants, attended weekly meetings, and actively participated in one Atlanta-area comité. The comité I regularly attended was organized by Doña Julia, a woman who dedicated countless hours to GLAHR, taught herself how to read as an adult, and made delicious *pozole*, a traditional Mexican hominy stew. Julia held weekly meetings in her apartment, where three-to-six neighbors would join us to hear Doña Julia explain what she learned at the weekly GLAHR meeting. By being involved in Julia's comité and GLAHR, I entered Atlanta's world of immigrant rights activism and met organization leaders, undocumented immigrants, health providers, policy makers, and others who contributed to the research that has resulted in this book. I owe these activists a debt that cannot be repaid. As anthropologist Sarah Horton has described, engaged anthropological work is an unfinished type of work in progress, and a book is one part of fulfilling an ongoing commitment to engaged scholarship and solidarity (2016b, 11).

BOOK STRUCTURE

This book is organized in seven proceeding chapters. Following an understanding of immigrant policing as a form of health policy, chapter 1 provides a history of policies regarding immigrants' health in the United States, paying specific attention to their exclusion from health services. Chapter 1 also contextualizes how immigrant policing fits into a broader matrix of race-based immigration policies. Extending the discussion about race-based exclusions, I also summarize the theoretical underpinnings of this book, drawing specifically from theories of biopolitics and citizenship. These theories allow for examining how immigrant policing regimes produce a type of fear-based governance in an effort to fashion undocumented immigrants into self-reliant neoliberal citizens who will not make demands on the state, which I expand on in chapter 3. In chapter 2, I examine how policy makers conceptualize immigration laws such as HB 87 and discuss some of the challenges with conducting a multi-sited ethnography, such as recruiting legislators who champion anti-immigrant policies. I further describe how HB 87's lawsuit provision inspired vigilant government agency-watching by at least one anti-undocumented immigrant activist and his organization. Findings from chapter 2 underscore challenges in studying governmental power and suggest that immigrant policing efforts are a way for policy makers to devise efficient techniques of power that manage entire populations.

Demonstrating how immigrant policing regimes manage populations through fear, I detail in chapter 3 how fear of encountering an increasingly localized immigration regime has resulted in some undocumented immigrants avoiding or finding alternative sources for care, revealing short-term implications on health and long-term concerns over a shadow medical system that obfuscates larger concerns related to unequal access to care and the impact of law enforcement.[13] Chapter 4 extends the discussion of immigrant policing impacting health into interpersonal realms, paying specific attention to intimate partner violence and concerns over parent-child separation. Findings from this chapter point to how immigrant policing can operate within home spaces and destabilize immigrant communities from within intimate settings such as the home. By focusing on the interpersonal consequences of immigrant policing, I examine some of the gendered elements of immigration enforcement regimes and draw from theories of intersectionality to describe how immigrant policing contributes to social inequalities rooted in race, sex, gender, and sexual orientation. Paying specific attention to undocumented lesbian, gay, bisexual, transgender, and otherwise queer-identifying (LGBTQ+) immigrants, I also describe some of the problems with using family narratives to assert some immigrants' deservingness to remain in the country.

Shifting attention from undocumented immigrants, in chapter 5 I examine how immigrant policing affects health providers and how health providers respond to immigration laws directly challenging their professional authority. Providers in this chapter suggest how they resist efforts to advance immigrants' illegitimacy as patients, but may be forced into adopting the logics of market-based medicine that undergird the U.S. health system, highlighting how immigrant-policing regimes directly impact providers' clinical practices. In chapter 6[14], I describe the larger, systemic concerns related to immigrant policing that affect hospitals and potentially the overall medical safety net. Focusing on Grady Memorial Hospital in Atlanta, I describe how the area's large public hospital subsidizes private health care facilities that "dump" undocumented patients because immigrant policing efforts have given them a license to discriminate. I further discuss how patient dumping is complicated by the most recent U.S. health reform law, and show how sending undocumented patients to Grady from other hospitals reveals weaknesses within the U.S. health safety net. In chapter 7, I conclude the book with a discussion about immigration detention, provide suggestions for how to fight against harsh anti-immigration laws, and describe how other activist groups have been successful in fighting certain forms of state power.

Though this book implicates policy and police activity in poor health, it is not a thorough account of the numerous black and brown men, women, and trans residents of the United States who die at the hands of police officers every year. It is also not a sufficient account of how race-based policing operates in the United States, or the consequences of racially driven legislation and police practices. Activist movements like Black Lives Matter continue to show how police power can violently reinforce racial hierarchies and inequalities, and these movements are reminders of how racial injustice continues to demand activist, scholarly, and political action. In focusing on immigration enforcement policy and health, this ethnography provides additional examples of how policy and police activity converge and have deleterious consequences. Medical anthropologists have pointed to how police action can result in nuanced forms of harm, using the term "pathogenic law enforcement" (Bourgois and Schonberg 2009, 111–113) to describe the health-related consequences of police officer intervention with vulnerable populations, including undocumented immigrants (Alexander and Fernandez 2014). Pathogenic law enforcement, or as I call it, pathogenic policing, is an analytical frame that specifically indicts law, policy, and law enforcement agents in perpetuating poor health and health inequalities that fit into a larger rubric of health inequity shaped by race, gender, sexual orientation, immigration status, and other social markers of difference.

I am grateful for the friendships that developed out of conducting the research for this book, and for the privilege of being able to write some of the thoughts, feelings, reactions, and lived experiences of people I met and who have to live with the consequences of immigrant policing. As I was finishing the research for this book, there appeared to be political efforts to provide undocumented immigrants reprieve from deportation, and at one point, the end of the Secure Communities program had been announced (Linthicum 2014). However, after the 2016 election of Donald Trump as the forty-fifth president of the United States, Secure Communities was reinstated, and numerous immigrant rights organizations feared what might happen to the communities where they work. Accordingly, immigrant policing efforts continue to demand attention. Existing and past policies aimed at governing immigrants through fear have had serious consequences that require action, as I show in the following chapters.

1 · HOW DID WE GET HERE?

Immigrant Policing in the United States

In 2012, protestors from the Cobb United for Change Coalition (CUCC) assembled in the central square in Marietta, a northern suburb of Atlanta in Cobb County. Marietta is notable for what has been described as "one of the most infamous outbursts of anti-Semitic feeling in the United States" (Dinnerstein 2008, xv): the 1915 lynching of Leo Frank, a Jewish man who moved from New York and was convicted of a crime based on dubious evidence. Marietta is also known among some immigrant rights activists for its anti-immigrant fervor because it is synonymous with Cobb County sheriff Neil Warren, who prides himself on being one of the "toughest sheriffs on illegal immigration" (Cobb County Sheriff's Office 2015) in the United States. At the rally in the square, CUCC members condemned HB 87 and called on Warren to end aggressive immigrant policing tactics like racial profiling. Anti-immigrant counterprotestors, some of whom brought guns for intimidation, also assembled outside the square. "See this picture," Joaquín, a local activist in his forties said as he handed me a folded newspaper he retrieved from his car. "This is them—they brought guns to the protest to show us they would shut us up."

Anti-immigrant intimidation was nothing new to activists like Joaquín. His friend Rich, a white, U.S.-born, self-identified ally to undocumented immigrants and fellow CUCC member, had been receiving threatening phone calls and letters depicting a man hanging from a tree since 2008. The threats started when Rich criticized a local bar for featuring anti-immigrant signs as part of its décor and selling racist caricatures of then president Barack Obama. Rich's public commentaries in local media and involvement in immigrant rights organizations resulted in a Cobb County-based anti-immigrant group listing Rich's phone number and email address on its website. In 2011, after more public confrontations with anti-immigrant groups, Rich found his family dog dead on his doorstep. A local veterinarian determined the dog's death to be the result of blunt force trauma. To Rich, his dog's death represented the extent to which anti-immigrant sentiment can go. "It shows the hate against immigrants and anyone who defends them," Rich explained. Months into my fieldwork, I learned about additional threatening emails Rich received, some of which featured disturbing and overtly racist language. I asked another local activist about why he thought Rich did not talk more about these threats. "He has to be careful about this stuff," the activist told me. "They slaughtered the man's dog on his front porch, for god's sake! This is some scary white supremacist stuff."

The anti-immigrant sentiment Joaquín saw on display in Marietta, and Rich witnessed through violent threats and actions, is not unique among anti-immigrant groups in Georgia. On the contrary, anti-immigrant sentiment has directly shaped U.S. policy. For example, on January 27, 2017, shortly after taking the oath of President of the United States, Donald Trump issued Executive Order 13769, more commonly referred to as "the Muslim ban, " which limited travel into the United States from countries with majority Muslim populations.[1] Former presidential hopeful Bernie Sanders called the order "racist and anti-Islamic," pointing to its discriminatory basis (Jordain Carney 2017). Donald Trump campaigned on enacting a Muslim ban and reducing immigration; and in his announcement that he was running for president, he referred to Mexican immigrants as "rapists" (Washington Post Staff 2015). But long before the election and the candidacy of Donald Trump, U.S. immigration policies were preoccupied with race and specifically conflated notions of race with immigrants' health status and their purported likelihood of needing governmental assistance. Nationally, immigrant policing efforts have squarely operated on racial difference, as demonstrated in Maricopa County, Arizona, where Sheriff Joe Arpaio persistently racially profiled Latinx drivers, leading him to defy the court orders to cease racial profiling (Associated Press 2016).[2] Accordingly, the numerous health-related impacts of immigrant policing that I describe in this book fit into a larger context of immigration policies that, on the basis of race, regulate immigrants and restrict their rights to social services like publicly funded health care.

In the United States, race-based exclusions have a history of informing immigrants' access to social services, including health care. It is no coincidence that the estimated eleven-to-twelve million undocumented immigrants living in the United States account for one out of four people of the uninsured population (Garfield and Damico 2016; Passel, Cohn, and Gonzalez-Barrera 2013; Sommers 2013; Zuckerman, Waidmann, and Lawton 2011; Livingston 2009), and as anthropologist Jason De León (2015) has argued, some immigration policies are deliberately implicated in immigrants' deaths. In an attempt to justify why undocumented immigrants should be denied access to certain health services, immigration critics frequently argue that undocumented immigrants "steal" public services, including health care. Contrary to such arguments, however, undocumented immigrants are *less* likely to use publicly funded services than their citizen or documented counterparts (Ortega et al. 2007). Furthermore, as I show in this chapter, numerous policies in the United States make it as difficult as possible for undocumented immigrants to access any type of health service, which may contribute to immigrants getting sicker the longer they live in the United States.

Immigrants typically arrive in the United States healthier than their native-born counterparts, but their health declines over time as a result of their living and working conditions and experiencing the effects of living in a racially stratified society (Himmelgreen et al. 2007; Antecol and Bedard 2006; Abraído-Lanza, Chao, and Flórez 2005; McEwen 2004). In many cases, immigrants' poor health is directly linked to their labor. As a result of working in the construction and agricultural industries, for example, some undocumented immigrants face serious occupational health risks that result in disproportionately high rates of injury, chronic disease, and disability compared with U.S. citizens (see, for example, Arcury and Quandt 2007). Immigrant policing efforts are another layer of social conditions that harm undocumented immigrants' health.

Despite these health burdens, undocumented immigrants are unable to participate in most publicly financed health programs. They typically lack employer-provided insurance and often engage in low-wage work that constrains their ability to purchase health insurance (American Nurses Association 2010; Kaiser Commission on Facts 2008; Okie 2007). Contemporary examples of exclusion from (and limited access to) medical care, oral health care, and mental health services have been well documented, and such exclusions can contribute to lasting health disparities and decreased quality of life (Kline 2012, 2010; Castañeda, Carrion et al. 2010; Horton and Barker 2010; Escobar, Constanza, and Gara 2009; Arcury and Quandt 2007). Exclusion from social and health services has an established history, as do policies that regulate immigrants' lives around social devices such as race. As anthropologists have noted, policy is a tool people use to organize themselves (Shore and Wright 1997, 6) and an instrument of political power that can drive ideologies and inequalities (Wedel et al. 2005). In this chapter, I examine the policies of exclusion that prevent undocumented immigrants from obtaining publicly financed care and situate those policies within the historical trajectory of race-based immigrant exclusion.

WHO ARE GEORGIA'S UNDOCUMENTED IMMIGRANTS?

A stroll through Midtown Atlanta feels like a walk in many other large U.S. cities. Skyscrapers flank wide sidewalks punctuated with trees, and car horns blare as frustrated motorists try to escape clogged streets and make their way to even more congested highways. Spread across three neighborhoods, Atlanta's skyline has more high-rises than any other city in the southeastern United States, except for Miami (Emporis, 2019a). Some of the nation's tallest buildings, including one of the top 20, are in Atlanta (Emporis 2019b), evidencing the city's status as a metropolis. The Atlanta area is home to some of the United States' major corporations, including Coca-Cola, Delta Airlines, Turner Broadcasting System, Home Depot,

United Parcel Service, and Rubbermaid. And as in other major U.S. cities, the Atlanta economy could not survive without immigrant labor fueling construction, hospitality, and tourist industries.

In 1999, Damián, a twenty-year-old from Guatemala, came to the United States to visit a friend during a college break. While staying at his friend's house for three months, Damián decided to get a part-time job to have some spending money. When his three-month stay in Georgia was coming to an end, Damián decided to extend his time in the United States, this time for three years instead of months, so he could work and send money to his brothers and parents. When he was twenty-one, his plans changed. "My father died," Damián said, his smile fading from his youthful face. With the somber news of his father's death, Damián decided to stay in the United States indefinitely. "I was the only one old enough to work and send money to my family; I was the only one who could take care of them." From 1999 to 2003, Damián lived in Atlanta without any trouble from police. Around 2005, however, Damián felt the area began to change. "All these laws started passing," he explained, and he noticed police started aggressively setting up checkpoints in Latinx neighborhoods. Like many immigrants in Atlanta, Damián works in construction. When we met, his younger brothers had recently moved to Atlanta, and on occasion, his sixteen-year-old brother would come to GLAHR meetings.

Damián's story of moving to Atlanta in the late 1990s matches those of many other immigrants in the area. As historian Mary Odem (2008) has described, Atlanta's immigrant community grew along with rapid economic transformation. During the 1990s, the Atlanta area added more jobs than any other metropolitan area in the country except for Dallas, Texas, and as white and black workers moved into salaried or higher-skilled jobs, immigrants filled needed laborer positions (Odem 2008, 108). From 1980 to 2005, immigrants from around the globe moved to Atlanta, and the total immigrant population in the area increased by more than 1,000 percent, transforming the city's economic, cultural, and political landscape (Odem 2008, 108). It is estimated that more than 700,000 Asian, European, and African immigrants live in Atlanta, including nearly 550,000 Latinx immigrants, the majority of whom are from Mexico (Brown and Lopez 2013; Wilson and Singer 2011).

Latinx immigrants in Atlanta settled in suburban neighborhoods in surrounding counties like Cobb, rather than the urban core. This settlement pattern was different from those of other U.S. cities, and it occurred in part because of an affordable, older apartment and housing stock. As newly arriving Latinx immigrants settled along major thoroughfares such as Buford Highway, they transformed dead shopping malls and economically reinvigorated stagnant neighborhoods (Odem 2008, 115–116). As Odem explains, in many cases, immigrants shared houses and apartments with family members, friends, and acquaintances from countries where they emigrated, and this type of suburban settlement created new racial tensions in the metro area, as Joaquín's account of the intimidation effort in Marietta Square suggests. Further, Atlanta's suburbs have a history of racial segregation that county governments have maintained through real estate and transportation policies like prohibiting public transportation stops in certain municipalities. Many of these governments responded to an influx of brown bodies by more closely enforcing certain housing codes and passing ordinances designed to discourage immigrant settlement, like English-signage requirements and day-laborer bans (Odem 2008). As Georgia politician Stacey Abrams explains in the next chapter, elected officials used racial tensions to promote anti-immigrant legislation and aggressive policing tactics. The relationship between immigration and race is nothing new, however, and certainly not unique to Georgia. Rather, race and immigration have been intimately linked in national policy.

RACE, IMMIGRATION, AND FEDERAL POLICIES OF EXCLUSION

In the United States, immigration policies and attitudes about immigrants have historically been shaped by labor needs and perceptions of immigrants' racial differences (Fairchild 2004; Calavita 2000; Chang 2000). For example, during the nineteenth century, the federal government and railroad employers welcomed Chinese immigrants to work on the Central Pacific Railroad as a much-needed and cheap labor source (Calavita 2000). When the railroad was completed and an economic recession hit in the 1870s, however, work opportunities became scarce and anti-immigrant rhetoric surged. Racist constructions of Chinese immigrants as "peculiar" and "racially inferior" became part of official political discourse (Calavita 2000). White labor groups pushed for anti-Chinese legislation, and in 1882, declaring that "the Chinese are peculiar in every aspect," Congress passed the Chinese Exclusion Act, banning Chinese laborers from entering the United States for ten years (Calavita 2000; Chang 2000).[3] Although policies excluding immigrants from the United States have existed since the 1700s (Feagin 1997), it was not until this period that immigrant exclusion merged with labor needs and racial notions of otherness.[4] The Chinese Exclusion Act was thus one of the first federal immigration laws and initiated a series of regulations based on conflated notions of race and national origin that continued throughout the twentieth century (De Genova 2004).

As the federal government took additional measures to control immigration, immigration laws increasingly focused on labor needs, race, and immigrants' health status. When Congress passed the 1891 Immigration Act, it assigned the federal government authority to control and centralize immigration processes. The act created the Office of the Superintendent of Immigration (OSI), housed within the Treasury Department, which oversaw all immigration activities along the

Canadian and Mexican borders and at Ellis Island. Key tasks for the OSI included inspecting newly arriving immigrants, and OSI staff were given the task of denying entry to any person who "would become a public charge," was convicted of a felony or crimes of "moral turpitude," practiced polygamy, or suffered from a "loathsome or a dangerous contagious disease" (Immigration Act of 1891, Pub. L. No. 51-551, 26 Stat. 1084a). "Loathsome diseases" included infectious eye diseases, fungal, parasitic, and sexually transmitted infections, tuberculosis, and mental conditions defined as insanity, idiocy, and epilepsy (Fairchild 2004, 530). In 1903, the inspections broadened to physically examine immigrants for conditions that would make them more likely to depend on public assistance, including chronic conditions such as heart disease, and conditions such as poor eyesight, varicose veins, "poor physique," and pregnancy (Fairchild 2004). Immigrants considered undesirable as workers or belonging to "inferior races" were denied entry, and their exclusion was justified by such medical rationalizations (Fairchild 2004, 530). In this combined public health and immigration control enterprise, health and race were understood as inherently linked, which determined the desirability of immigrants being inspected.

Merged notions of race and health became more deeply entrenched in U.S. immigration laws with the passage of the Emergency Quota Law of 1921. The law established quotas that limited the number of immigrants who could enter the United States on the basis of conflated notions of racial inferiority and health status. One of the motivations for the law was to reduce the number of southern and eastern European immigrants entering the United States because they were considered racially inferior to northern Europeans and were described in the law as "abnormally twisted," "unassimilable," "filthy un-American" (Calavita 1996, 288–299). When the law was extended in 1924, it limited the number of immigrants allowed to enter the United States to 150,000 people per year, restricting immigration to only 2 percent of each racial category recorded in the 1890 census: a deliberate effort to favor immigration from northern European countries and construct American whiteness in a specific fashion. Such restrictions were designed to drastically limit the number of Jewish, Italian, and eastern and southern European immigrants who were considered "non-white" and thus physically, intellectually, and genetically inferior (Fairchild 2004, 5). The national origin system favoring northern and western Europeans over southern and eastern Europeans was abolished in 1965, but the quotas put in place by the 1924 law effectively changed immigration patterns in the United States in the early twentieth century.

As European immigrants were gradually considered "white" and not racially different from one another, U.S. immigration policies slowly changed. Immigration laws also changed to keep up with labor demands. When immigration levels continued to fall during World War II, the United States experienced a labor shortage, and in what immigration scholar Nicholas De Genova calls "a dramatic reversal of the mass deportations of the 1930s" (2004, 164), the United States federal government loosened immigration policy, granting entry to Mexican and Chinese workers (Fairchild 2004). Labor needs were so acute in some industries, such as agriculture, that the federal government began importing laborers from Mexico through an agreement known as the Bracero Program, which promised certain housing conditions and wages to farmworkers.

The Bracero Program began in 1942 and was continually renewed and expanded until its termination in 1964 (De Genova 2004). Like European immigrants arriving through Ellis Island, Mexican agricultural workers who entered the United States through the program underwent health inspections. U.S. and Mexican public health doctors physically inspected Bracero workers for health conditions such as tuberculosis, "venereal disease," and physical signs suggesting they would be unfit for agricultural labor (Hoffman 2006, 239). Although Congress officially canceled the Bracero Program after more than twenty years of operation, agricultural labor migration from Mexico to the United States continued. Mexican immigrants and U.S. employers had well-established relationships, and instead of ceasing movement and labor arrangements, the program's cancellation led to increases in underground, "illegal" immigration. As immigration and legal scholar Kitty Calavita notes, "With the end of the program, the employment of Mexican labor went underground as the guest workers of one era became the illegal immigrants of the next" (1996, 289).

Shortly after the Bracero Program ended, Congress passed the Immigration and Nationality Act (INA) in 1965, which abolished racial restrictions of the national origins quota system but simultaneously implemented new restrictions focused on immigrants from the Western Hemisphere (De Genova 2004). The INA amendments specifically capped the number of immigrants from Mexico and any other Western Hemisphere country at 120,000 people (Massey and Pren 2012; De Genova 2004), even though the number of Mexicans entering the United States as part of a migrant farm labor circuit averaged nearly 500,000 per year by the late 1950s (Massey and Pren 2012). In amending the INA, Congress mirrored racial quotas for immigrants set in the 1920s but focused on Mexican immigrants and immigrants from Latin America and dramatically reduced the number of Mexicans eligible for legal residency (Massey and Pren 2012; De Genova 2004). Just as eastern and southern Europeans were once restricted from entry and residency, now so were Mexican immigrants.

While labor demands have certainly played an important role in U.S. immigration policy, so too have notions of racial difference. The racial exclusion of immigrant groups operated on perceptions of immigrants' overall biological inferiority, including their health status (Fairchild 2004; Braun 2002). Notions of racial difference and perceived inferior health status resulted in U.S. Public Health Service workers physically inspecting immigrants before they could enter the country, and health-related anxieties continue to be a basis for denying immigrants' entry into the United States. Racialized notions of disease and social utility have driven immigration policy (Braun 2002) and have also become articulated in financial terms, as demonstrated by concerns over unhealthy immigrants becoming a "public charge" after they enter the United States (Sainsbury 2006; Fairchild 2004). But why would a government pass immigration policies based on notions of racial otherness? The United States has a substantial history of policies based on race, but why might immigration policies also focus on race?

RACE, IMMIGRATION, AND POWER

As I described in the introduction, I examine immigration enforcement policies and their numerous health-related consequences. I examine policy as a type of power, and as I have already noted, I borrow from philosopher Michel Foucault's work on how power is applied over life and over a population—what he called "biopower" (1978, 140). As Foucault demonstrates, race and exercises of power, like legislation or policy, have an important relationship and can demonstrate how groups of people can be managed.

In examining how power is applied over life, Foucault argues that mechanisms of power have changed significantly over time. He specifically notes that around the seventeenth and eighteenth centuries, power mechanisms were designed to "control," "order," and "optimize" life and "make it grow" rather than "destroy" it (1978, 136). As part of this power over life, Foucault describes what he calls "biopolitics," a type of power focused on the population (1978, 139). The emergence of this new technology of power that focused on humans as a species rather than individual human bodies represents the beginning of managing human "races" (Foucault 2003, 242). In managing human beings as a race or population, biopolitical technologies focus on a population's "vital" characteristics related to life, such as morbidity due to endemic and epidemic disease, mortality, birth rates, health status, and fertility (N. Rose 2007; Foucault 2003). In other words, biopolitics can be understood as a form of power concerned with the population instead of individuals (Foucault 2003, 246).[5] As a form of power concerned with population-level interventions and organizations, biopolitics includes specific technologies designed to subdivide human beings based on categorization schemes, such as race. Race, then, can be understood as one type of biopolitical technology since it is a tool to intervene on the entire human population and organize or categorize it. Additionally, racism, as Foucault defines it, is a process of separating groups within a population for fragmentation, hierarchization, determining superiority and inferiority, and otherwise subdividing populations established through biological frames (2003, 255).

According to Foucault, racism has two specific functions: to fragment a population and to create a biological relationship based on survival and success, which can ultimately justify death through the life and success of another race (2003,

255–256). In other words, racism is a way to justify why some populations should be successful and others not, and to a greater extreme, why some should live and others should die. In addition to the literal meanings of life and death, this idea can be extended to a metaphorical sense—that racism can justify investment in some lives and not others so that one group flourishes and another figuratively "dies" because of a perceived racial inferiority (Kline 2017).

How might immigration policy in the United States relate to biopolitics and race? First and foremost, immigration policy has been rooted in notions of racial otherness, as demonstrated by the various policies that resulted in immigrants being denied entry or excluded from the country based on perceptions of racial inferiority. Racial difference informed U.S. immigration policy, making such policy a biopolitical technology. In the early twentieth century, efforts to keep allegedly "filthy" immigrants out of the United States were ways to optimize and invest in the existing U.S. population, at the expense of denying entry to some immigrants. Foucault might consider such an effort to fall under what he refers to as a "race-war logic," or using racial difference to ensure the success and thriving of one race at the expense of others.[6] As anthropologist Mae Ngai has argued, race-based quotas from early immigration policies were partly informed by eugenicists' reports of potential "degradation to the white race" (2004, 24). Such anxieties directly informed race-based immigration quotas created in the early twentieth century, which established what Ngai calls "a global racial and national hierarchy that favored some immigrants over others" (2004, 3). Favoring immigrants with qualities associated with "whiteness," specifically, has endured over time. Anthropologists Sarah Horton and Aihwa Ong, for example, have both described how immigration policies and immigrants' reception into the United States continue to be associated with perceived qualities that are aligned with "whiteness" (Horton 2004; Ong 1996, 1995).[7] Those qualities have typically included preconceived notions of entrepreneurship and economic self-sufficiency, as demonstrated by policies preoccupied with preventing racially othered immigrants from entering the country because of fears of them becoming "public charges."

While immigration laws have changed in the United States, the vestiges of prior policies remain. As policy makers described to me (in chapter 2), economic rationales continue to inform anti-immigrant legislation in Georgia, specifically. Additionally, although the national origins quota system has been abolished, concerns about immigrants overusing public services that were initially conflated with race, and anxieties about immigrants being "public charges," persist in contemporary U.S. immigration legislation. Starting with the first federal public health program, the Social Security Act of 1965, anxieties about immigrants' use of publicly funded programs have informed how some immigrants continue to be excluded from health services. Excluding some immigrant groups from social services is a way of reforming historical race-based exclusions that shift from wholesale exclusion from entering the country to being denied social services.

A HISTORY OF EXCLUSION FROM HEALTH SERVICES

In the United States, there are few options for undocumented immigrants who need health care. The U.S. health care system operates on a market-based model (Rylko-Bauer and Farmer 2002; and see, for example, Maskovsky 2000), and the majority of people finance their care through health insurance obtained through their employers (Barnett and Vornovitsky 2016). There are limited publicly funded health programs, and undocumented immigrants are typically ineligible for those programs. When they need care, undocumented immigrants are often relegated to hospital emergency rooms, charitable clinics, or community health centers, which provide primary care for indigent patients but are insufficiently funded to meet the needs of all medically underserved populations (Shin et al. 2013; Rosenbaum et al. 2010). Exclusion from the mainstream health care system undermines overall public health goals, but this form of exclusion is historically rooted in the creation of the Social Security Act of 1965—the nation's oldest health entitlement program.

The Social Security Act of 1965 created Medicare and Medicaid to serve individuals over sixty-five and low-income families, respectively. Despite political efforts and proposals to shrink, defund, and abolish these programs, they remain critical health care policies for millions of U.S. residents. Medicare alone provides benefits for more than 55 million people in the United States (Kaiser Family Foundation 2015), or 17 percent of the entire population. Since their creation, eligibility for Medicare and Medicaid has required U.S. citizenship or authorized entry into the United States. As a result, legal permanent residents were allowed to participate in the programs, whereas undocumented immigrants were not (Kaiser Commission on Facts 2008). In creating these restrictions, the Social Security Act of 1965 was the first federal effort to exclude undocumented immigrants from specific types of health care. By focusing on denying entitlements to undocumented immigrants, the provisions created in the Social Security Act of 1965 marked a shift in federal legislation and departed from previous systems of exclusion based on race and health status, which targeted immigrants *before* entering the country. Unlike previous forms of immigrant exclusion, such as the Emergency Quota Law, the Social Security Act created a new system of exclusion based on immigration status that affected immigrants who had *already* entered the United States instead of those who were attempting to enter. This shift was the first federal effort to exclude undocumented immigrants from specific health services, which had reverberating influences on future social service and health policies. Because of the precedent set by the Social Security Act, undocumented immigrants continue to be restricted from receiving publicly funded services unless they experience medical emergencies, or in the case of women, are pregnant, which I discuss later in this chapter.

Despite being denied publicly funded health care by the Social Security Act of 1965, undocumented immigrants are still eligible for publicly funded health services through emergency rooms.[8] In the United States, emergency room practices are governed in part by the Emergency Medical Treatment and Active Labor Act (EMTALA) of 1985. Under EMTALA, hospital emergency rooms are required to treat patients who have emergent conditions regardless of diagnosis, race, ability to pay, national origin, physical ability, or any other characteristic. The law was passed to stop hospitals from transferring indigent patients from one hospital to another—a process known as "patient dumping" (Lee 2004)—before they were medically stable. Before EMTALA, any person unable to pay for care, including undocumented immigrants, could be denied care from a hospital emergency room, and hospitals throughout the United States dumped patients who were unable to pay, had existing medical conditions, or were pregnant (Lee 2004). Although EMTALA effectively allowed for all patients to receive services through emergency rooms, the law has not put an end to all forms of patient dumping, as I describe in chapter 6. Nevertheless, EMTALA formalized an effective "right" to emergency health services for all populations (Lee 2004), regardless of citizenship status.

To financially assist hospitals taking large numbers of uninsured patients they were obligated to stabilize, Congress created the Disproportionate Share Hospital (DSH) program, which increased Medicaid payments to hospitals with large numbers of uninsured and Medicaid patients (Warner 2012). Together, EMTALA and DSH provide a way for undocumented immigrants to receive publicly financed care, but only in emergency situations. With the passage of the United States' most recent health reform law, the Patient Protection and Affordable Care Act (ACA), however, DSH funding and emergency care for undocumented immigrants may be threatened (see chapter 6). Moreover, immigrant policing efforts disrupt EMTALA and DSH processes in ways that threaten care for all indigent populations. Even though undocumented immigrants ostensibly have access to publicly financed health care through emergency rooms because of EMTALA and DSH, and despite lacking access to care through nearly all other channels, they are less likely than U.S.-born residents to seek care in emergency rooms (Pourat et al. 2014; Ku and Matani 2001). Indeed, as I noted earlier in this chapter, undocumented immigrants use fewer health resources than documented or citizen populations, but politicians and some U.S. residents nevertheless accuse them of being "drains" on the public health care system.

The rhetoric of being a public charge that informed immigration concerns in the early twentieth century continued throughout the 1980s and 1990s with neoliberal welfare reforms. These reforms championed neoliberal economic ideals such as shrinking the size of government, emphasizing individual reasonability, and promoting market-based principles over all aspects of life (Harvey 2007; Ong 2006; Hyatt 2001; Wacquant 2001; Maskovsky 2000; Schneider 1999). Neoliberal ideals directly shaped immigration laws, including the 1986 "amnesty" legislation Ronald Reagan signed: the Immigration Reform and Control Act (IRCA).[9] When IRCA passed, it provided a pathway to citizenship for some undocumented immigrants, but it made citizenship contingent on proving immigrants had never received federal public benefits such as Medicaid (Huang 2008). IRCA's restrictions resulted in confusion among some immigrants who received state-level assistance for which they were eligible and continues to deter some immigrants from using state or federal benefits for themselves or their eligible U.S.-citizen children (Huang 2008). Further restricting undocumented immigrants' eligibility to obtain health services were the Personal Responsibility and Work Opportunity Reconciliation Act (PRWORA) and the Illegal Immigration Reform and Immigrant Responsibility Act (IIRIRA), which passed in 1996.

Synonymous with "welfare reform" of the 1990s, PRWORA remains one of the most sweeping legislative changes to social services in U.S. history and resulted in new policies emphasizing neoliberal notions of personal responsibility. As with other neoliberal reforms, discourses surrounding PRWORA cast the nation's poorest populations and racial minorities as incompliant with market-based expectations of individual responsibility. This rhetorical scapegoating suggested that because poor and minority populations were purportedly irresponsible, they would abuse social services, be dependent on welfare, and use children to gain access to entitlement programs (O'Daniel 2008; Maskovsky 2005; Chang 2000; L. Chavez 1997). Lawmakers lumped together immigrants with poor, racial minorities who they alleged would abuse federal programs, and specifically wrote into the legislation that public benefits were an "incentive" for unauthorized immigration (Kullgren 2003; United States Congress 1996) despite evidence to the contrary. By reducing federal welfare expenditures and thereby allegedly ending so-called cultures of dependency among the poor and "removing incentives for illegal immigration," PRWORA promised to save $54.1 billion over six years, half of which resulted from cutting services to immigrants (Fairchild 2004; Ellwood and Ku 1998). Overall, PRWORA's cost savings were made possible by creating new eligibility restrictions on authorized immigrants and their children (Huang, Stella, and Ledsky 2006; Fairchild 2004; Ku and Matani 2001).

Before PRWORA, citizens and authorized immigrants shared equal access to public programs. Changes in PRWORA, however, divided all immigrants from citizens and further subdivided immigrants into qualified and nonqualified aliens, making residency, citizenship, and length of time in the United States requirements for receiving certain entitlements (Viladrich 2012). On a state level, PRWORA gave states nearly total control of welfare programs, which allowed for some state and local governments to create more benefits to undocumented populations (Marrow 2012), but simultaneously created more stringent work requirements and limits to receiving benefits (Ellwood and Ku 1998).

Similar to federal benefit restrictions for authorized immigrants created by PRWORA, IIRIRA created new restrictions to social services for undocumented immigrants. The welfare provisions of IIRIRA extended beyond health services and specifically barred undocumented immigrants from receiving any type of federal benefit, including nutritional and housing program benefits, work and professional licenses, contracts, disability benefits, and other forms of assistance. The law also made it more challenging for authorized immigrants to receive public benefits after a five-year residency requirement and further strengthened the "public charge" exclusions created in earlier immigration laws (K. Johnson 2009; Clark 2008). Under changes made in IIRIRA, when applying for benefits, an immigrant must include a sponsor, friend, or family member whose income is included in calculating benefit eligibility (Huang 2008). These restrictions responded to public and political accusations of undocumented immigrants using state resources, demonstrating how economic justifications for limiting undocumented immigrants' social services informed provisions of PRWORA and IIRIRA. Together, IIRIRA and PRWORA have resulted in decreased usage of social services such as Medicaid among some immigrants eligible for services owing to confusion about eligibility and other factors (Hagan et al. 2003). As a result, some immigrants who are eligible for Medicaid services in some locations have found alternate strategies to receiving care (Hagan et al. 2003). Like IRCA, then, IIRIRA ultimately set expectations and altered some immigrants' behaviors. These policies and their consequences underscore how policy can have hidden health-related consequences and also create sets of expectations for some populations.

In addition to restricting undocumented immigrants' ability to receive public benefits, IIRIRA established numerous provisions concerning border enforcement, stiffer penalties for smuggling and documentation fraud, changes in deportation proceedings, employer sanctions for hiring undocumented immigrants, and changes regarding refugees and asylum seekers (Fragomen 1997). The law also amended the INA by adding section 287(g), a program in which the federal government grants local police permission to enforce immigration laws, as I later describe. Components of PRWORA and IIRIRA demonstrate underlying neoliberal logics of self-reliance that informed the legislation and included immigration in their scope (Sainsbury 2006). Furthermore, they exemplify how economic concerns become conflated with racialized notions of immigrants' otherness that have resulted in the exclusion of undocumented immigrants from social services. This form of exclusion has been further codified in health reform efforts, including the ACA.

In 2009, Joe Wilson, U.S. representative for South Carolina, broke congressional decorum when he interrupted President Barack Obama's address to Congress. In his address, Obama laid out his proposal for health care reform and what would eventually become the ACA. He further responded to the myth that the ACA would provide health insurance to undocumented immigrants. Responding to Obama's assertion, Wilson pointed to the president and shouted "You lie!" twice. In his assessment of Wilson's outburst, anthropologist Josiah Heyman (2009) pointed out that the costs of caring for undocumented immigrants are relatively low and that the health of everyone, regardless of citizenship, is interconnected. Heyman argued that such a heated debate about undocumented immigrants receiving health services is directly linked to assumptions about them being undeserving of health services because of their method of entry into the United States. Anthropologists have shown in a number of global settings that undocumented immigrants' exclusion from health entitlements often hinges on assessments of their deservingness of social services, and the United States is no exception (Castañeda 2012; Viladrich 2012; Willen 2012, 2011; Goldade 2009; Yoo 2008).

Joe Wilson's outburst revealed tensions about undocumented immigrants' assumed lack of deservingness of publicly funded health care, and how immigrants are considered an "other" based race and immigration status. When the ACA passed, it continued to prohibit undocumented immigrants from receiving Medicaid (Sommers 2013; Warner 2012; Zuckerman, Waidmann, and Lawton 2011) and further prohibited undocumented immigrants from purchasing certain types of health insurance with their own funds (Cartwright 2011, 479). As I describe in chapter 6, the ACA had more indirect impacts on undocumented immigrants because it reduced DSH funds that reimburse hospitals for providing care to undocumented patients.

The ACA was one of two major health reform efforts in the United States since the creation of Medicare and Medicaid. Before the ACA, President Bill Clinton and First Lady Hillary Clinton attempted sweeping reforms to the U.S. health care system with little success. Although a comprehensive reform was unsuccessful, a smaller health care initiative focusing on children passed in 1997 (Oberlander and Lyons 2009). The program, State Children's Health Insurance Program, now the Children's Health Insurance Program (CHIP), expanded Medicaid to children in low-income families that otherwise earned too much to qualify for Medicaid. Since eligibility focuses on children, U.S.-citizen children with undocumented parents can participate in the program (Kaiser Commission on Facts 2006). Despite children's eligibility, however, some undocumented immigrant parents may not enroll their children in CHIP or take their CHIP-enrolled children to providers because of fears of being reported to immigration authorities (Castañeda and Melo 2014; Huang, Stella, and Ledsky 2006; Kullgren 2003; Ku and Matani 2001; Baumeister and Hearst 1999).

In providing health insurance to children, CHIP also allows for pregnant undocumented women to receive prenatal care. This was not written into the law or developed later through altruistic notions of providing care to all populations; rather, it was an effort to intervene on behalf of a potential unborn U.S. citizen. Prenatal care for undocumented women provided through CHIP only occurred after the Centers for Medicare and Medicaid Services changed the definition of "child" to include unborn children, effectively granting personhood to fetuses for treatment purposes and providing CHIP benefits to fetuses carried by undocumented women (Huang 2008). Access to health services for pregnant undocumented immigrant women was thus the consequence of a gendered policy valuing an unborn body that would be granted political citizenship by virtue of being born in the United States.

Overall, the policies I have described here have sent a symbolic message to some immigrants that they do not "belong" in U.S. society and should not attempt to use services that are accessible to, and the right of, other residents. In some circumstances, such as providing Medicaid to pregnant women for prenatal care, rationales for care are linked to U.S. citizenship and national belonging. However, citizenship encompasses more than national identity and place of birth. As I described in the introduction, the notion of citizenship describes how populations make claims for political, social, and economic recognition, and includes ideas about rights and obligations (Isin and Turner 2002). Rather than being a narrowly defined legal relationship between a person and a government (Sassen 2002, 278), citizenship is instead a relationship among individuals, a group of individuals, the polity, and other actors entangled in a network of power relationships. Medical anthropologists who have explored the idea of citizenship have shown that some populations may assert citizenship claims as part of power relationships. For example, some vulnerable populations may draw on their suffering to demand social services, health care, and biomedical interventions (Nguyen 2008; Biehl 2009; Rose and Novas 2005; Petryna 2004). Conversely, logics of exclusion based on ideas of citizenship can influence who receives and who is denied medical care (Scheper-Hughes 2006; Wailoo, Livingston, and Guarnaccia 2006). Citizenship in its broadest form therefore includes notions of rights, entitlements, and sets of relationships.

Policies like PRWORA, IIRIRA, and the ACA help send a message about immigrants' rights and entitlements. Economically scapegoating immigrants, limiting authorized immigrants' access to social services, and barring undocumented immigrants from purchasing health insurance with their own funds are ways of articulating to immigrants that they are not as deserving of various sets of rights and entitlements as other populations. Adding to health policies that assert immigrants' undeservingness of sets of rights and entitlements, recent immigration policies have doubled down on historical forms of casting immigrants as racial others, specifically by incorporating elements of alleged criminal deviance.

RACIALIZED CRIMINALITY AND GOVERNING
IMMIGRANTS THROUGH CRIME

Undocumented immigrants' exclusion from publicly funded health services is an extension of broader policies of exclusion. As critical race theorists have argued, the U.S. legal system has historically played a role in upholding racial inequalities (Delgado and Stefancic 2012; Villenas and Deyhle 1999; Crenshaw 1995), and immigration laws are no exception. Immigration legislation has "framed" (Goffman 1974) undocumented immigrants as criminal, deviant "others" who should be denied access to health services and punished as lawbreakers (Viladrich 2012; Yoo 2008; Fujiwara 2005; Horton 2004; Becker, Beyene, and Ken 2000). Frames of criminality and immigrant illegality mask the structural, political, and economic forces contextualizing migration and simplify migration as an individual choice. Moreover, frames of criminality and illegality carry implicit racial assumptions that inform policy. For example, in 2010, Arizona governor Jan Brewer held a press conference about Arizona's then-new immigration enforcement law, the Support Our Law Enforcement and Safe Neighborhoods Act, Senate Bill (SB) 1070. As I noted in the introduction, the law granted police the authority to stop anyone they suspected of being an "illegal immigrant." At the press conference, a reporter questioned how law enforcement might determine immigration status, asking Brewer, "What criteria would you use to determine if someone is an 'illegal immigrant'? What does an 'illegal immigrant' look like?" After a pause and chuckle, the flustered governor responded, "I do not know what an illegal immigrant looks like." The exchange underscored one of the many problems with immigration enforcement regimes: that they reinforce racial profiling and merge "illegality" with race and ethnicity.

Immigration scholars have noted that undocumented immigrants' criminal otherness has become conflated with race, specifically through the use of the idea of "illegality," making illegality itself a racialized category (Hiemstra 2010; Heyman 2008; L. Chavez 2007; Willen 2007b; De Genova 2004). As Mae Ngai points out, the term "illegal alien" in particular is "associated with racism towards Mexicans and other Latinos and Latinas" (2004, xiv). The term "illegal immigrant" effectively criminalizes all "brown bodies" (Hiemstra 2010, 79) and carries implicit assumptions about social deviance that justify punitive measures as a way to purportedly "protect" other populations. This is highlighted by the large number of immigrants held in federal custody. Noncitizens comprise almost one-third of the federal prison population (despite accounting for only thirteen percent of the entire U.S. population), and immigration violations remain a focus for the federal government (Migration Policy Institute 2014; Kretsedemas and Brotherton 2004). Further, the racialized illegality of Mexicans, in particular, fueled xenophobic attitudes in conservative politics throughout the 1990s and to the present, as evident in Donald Trump's comments about Mexican immigrants and his promise to build a complete wall between the United States and Mexico. These and other xenophobic attitudes have guided proposals to end birthright citizenship and sparked nativist paranoia about a white "majority" losing political control to a nonwhite "minority" population (De Genova 2005, 67).

Although U.S. immigration and social service policies criminalizing immigrants through racial constructions have a long history (K. Johnson 2009; Calavita 2005; De Genova 2004; Fairchild 2004), recent discourses of immigrants' criminality informing social service policies began with neoliberal reforms such as IRCA and PRWORA (Horton 2014). Many of the debates shaping PRWORA and its immigration provisions constructed undocumented immigrants as "career criminals" who not only enter the United States through unauthorized means but also allegedly counterfeit U.S. documents, fail to pay taxes, and "steal" taxpayers' resources by using public entitlements (Viladrich 2012). These arguments have repeated themselves in the United States over time in numerous levels of government. For example, Donald Trump accused undocumented immigrants of being responsible for economic troubles in the United States despite evidence indicating otherwise (Shih 2017). More than ignoring data on undocumented immigrants' economic contributions to the United States, Trump's claims and similar arguments fail to acknowledge that "illegal immigration" is largely driven by labor demands and is related to U.S. policy.

As I have argued, immigration policies have served to construct undocumented immigrants as criminal, racial others. Racial constructions of immigrant illegality intensified after September 11, 2001 (Fairchild 2004), and increased policing and deportation efforts have been justified in a post–9/11 rationalization of national security (T. Miller 2005). The development of illegality as a racialized, criminally deviant status has allowed for greater proliferation of immigration enforcement laws that I focus on in this book and that directly affect the GLAHRiadores and other Latinx immigrants in Georgia, like Joaquín. These laws aim, as immigration scholars Jonathan Inda and Julie Dowling explain, to "govern undocumented immigrants through crime" or "make crime and punishment the institutional context in which efforts to guide the conduct of immigrants take place" (2013, 2).

GOVERNING IMMIGRANTS THROUGH CRIME: INTERIOR ENFORCEMENT

As immigrants in Atlanta are well aware, a number of policies have attempted to govern immigrants by attempting to effectively criminalize their everyday conduct (Kline 2017). Through a number of immigration enforcement laws, tasks such as driving, looking for work, obtaining housing, turning on utilities, taking children to school, going to a grocery store, or any other mundane daily activity have become a risk for arrest and deportation for undocumented immigrants, as Adelina frequently highlighted in GLAHR meetings. The transformation of everyday life into a series of risky activities that resulted in Esme's concern for her husband and subsequent call to the GLAHR hotline, was made possible primarily through multiple, overlapping immigration enforcement efforts. At the core of this over-lapping immigration enforcement regime are two federal laws: section 287(g) of the INA (1996) and Secure Communities (2008).

As I described in the introduction, under the U.S. federalist system, power is divided between a national federal government and state governments, but the federal government historically has a host of exclusive powers, including immigration. However, the federal government's sole authority over immigration has changed under section 287(g) of the INA. Under section 287(g), local police enter memorandums of agreement (MOAs) with ICE, the principal federal office charged with immigration matters.[10] Through these MOAs, local officers are dep-utized as federal immigration agents and are allowed to enforce federal immigra-tion laws.[11] Through 287(g), officers have the authority to inquire about immi-gration status, issue warrants for immigration status violations, and act on search warrants while conducting routine police activity "in the field," such as stopping drivers for moving violations like speeding or not having a functional taillight (Capps et al. 2007). By deputizing local police, 287(g) permits a type of local-ized immigration enforcement that extends powers traditionally given exclusively to federal authorities to everyday law enforcement agents. As a mechanism of local-ized immigrant policing, 287(g) works in concert with other state and federal laws to impact undocumented immigrants' health.

One of the policies that 287(g) works with is Secure Communities. Like the 287(g) program, Secure Communities is a federal immigration program that works on local levels. The program matches fingerprints from jail inmates with immi-gration databases to assess detainees' immigration status. If an arrestee's finger-print is matched with a fingerprint of a noncitizen, including a lawfully present resident (see, for example, Aguilasocho, Rodwin, and Ashar 2012), local police hold the detainee for forty-eight hours and ICE officials are notified of the detain-ee's presence. For example, using Esme and Alvaro's situation, if a local officer arrested Alvaro for driving without a license, he would be taken to a local jail where officers would take his fingerprints. Through the Secure Communities program, those fingerprints would be matched against federal databases to determine if Alvaro had any criminal history and to determine his immigration status. ICE would then have forty-eight hours to interview Alvaro, make a decision about his presence in the United States, and begin the deportation process. If ICE fails to collect immigrants after the forty-eight-hour hold period, police must release the detainee.

Secure Communities was created under the George W. Bush administration in 2008 and expanded under Barack Obama. It has drawn considerable criticism for its costs to local governments and for leading to the alleged wrongful impris-onment of at least one U.S. citizen.[12] The program was discontinued but replaced by a similar program in 2014, and ultimately returned on January 25, 2017, through an executive order by Donald Trump. Although Secure Communities is ostensibly designed to target dangerous criminals, numerous immigrants like Alvaro, who do nothing more than try to live their daily lives, get swept up in an aggressive deportation regime.

In addition to Secure Communities and 287(g), immigration enforcement laws that directly affect immigrants like Alvaro work together with other policies purportedly created for security purposes, such as the REAL ID Act. The act is a federal law that requires state governments to assess driver's license applicants' citizenship or immigration status before issuing licenses. The REAL ID Act ultimately restricts undocumented immigrants' ability to receive driver's licenses, rendering them vulnerable to arrest if they get behind the wheel of a car. Since cars are a necessary mode of transportation in the United States, restricting access to driver's licenses is a key component of the multilayered immigrant policing regime. Police can arrest anyone driving without a license, and once in jail, their fingerprints can be matched using the Secure Communities program and ICE can be notified to interview them. Combined, the REAL ID Act, 287(g), and Secure Communities create a federal policy climate where immigrants are governed through crime; simply driving to accomplish a mundane task becomes a potentially criminal act, and undocumented immigrants' routine lives become risky activities since driving increases the risk of deportability (Stuesse and Coleman 2014). In addition to federal statutes aiming to govern immigrants through crime, a growing number of state legislatures have passed immigration statutes, including Georgia.

IMMIGRATION LEGISLATION IN GEORGIA

In 2010, police at Kennesaw State University, one of Georgia's public universities with two campuses in Marietta, stopped one of the university's students, Jessica Colotl. Officers stopped Colotl for blocking traffic in a campus parking lot. When they asked her for a driver's license, Colotl, who came to the United States when she was eleven years old, was unable to produce one because she is undocumented. Campus police arrested Colotl, and she was turned over to immigration authorities through the 287(g) program. The arrest occurred one semester before Colotol was expected to graduate, and her arrest put Georgia in the national spotlight for its 287(g) agreements, although it was not the first state to enter 287(g) agreements or pass immigration-related statutes.

In recent years, a growing number of state legislatures, including Georgia's, have passed immigration statutes. Legislators have specifically focused on social services, including publicly funded health care, in explaining the rationale for state immigration laws, echoing historical forms of rejecting immigrants based on concerns about them being a "public charge." One of the earliest forerunners of contemporary state immigration laws targeting undocumented immigrants' use of social services was California's Proposition 187. The California law passed by voter referendum in 1995 and made undocumented immigrants ineligible for a wide array of public services, including education and health services (Colino 1995). Undocumented-immigrant children were barred from enrolling in public schools, school administrators were required to inspect children's immigration status, and undocumented patients were denied state-funded emergency care, prenatal care, and vaccinations (Calavita 1996, 291). As a result of the initiative, undocumented immigrants' utilization of social services such as health care and public education declined (Fairchild 2004; Berk et al. 2000). Although a federal court ultimately found the law to be unconstitutional, the legislation successfully crafted a message of exclusion for undocumented immigrants that reemerged in other state laws (see, for example, Calavita 1996).

Starting a deluge of immigration laws passing in the 2000s and 2010s, Arizona passed SB 1070 in 2010, adopting a new strategy of sending a message of exclusion to undocumented immigrants that centered on law enforcement and their purported criminality. SB 1070 mandates that immigrants carry immigration documents with them at all times and compels law enforcement officials to assess an individual's immigration status if they suspect the individual may be undocumented. Similar laws passed in Alabama, Georgia, Indiana, South Carolina, and Utah (Sacks 2012), and Mississippi was at one point expected to pass comparable legislation but did not (Sutton 2012). Other states also passed immigration-specific legislation, resulting in a total of 164 anti-immigrant laws passed in state legislatures in 2010 and 2011 alone (Gordon and Raja 2012).

Following examples from California's Proposition 187 and Arizona's SB 1070, in recent years, Georgia has passed a series of immigration laws restricting undocumented immigrants' access to social services, including welfare benefits and specific forms of education. When Colotl was arrested in Cobb County and referred to immigration authorities through the 287(g) program, her situation sparked local and national debate about undocumented immigrants being admitted into public universities and shed national light on the plight of undocumented youth. In Georgia, her story led some legislators to demand that Georgia universities check students' immigration status before admission, and this inspired the first drafts of legislation restricting undocumented immigrants' ability to attend certain Georgia universities. The Georgia Board of Regents, receiving pressure from the state legislature, banned undocumented students from Georgia's top universities. Education measures have continued to be debated and discussed in the legislature, including proposed laws to ban unauthorized students from all of Georgia's public universities and technical colleges (for example, HB 59 from legislative year 2012). As I describe in chapter 7, these measures have inspired education-oriented activism, giving rise to an "underground university," Freedom University, in which faculty from the University of Georgia offer free classes for undocumented immigrants.

In addition to restricting education for undocumented youth, Georgia passed a state law dramatically augmenting the significance of driving without a license. Under Georgia law SB 350 (2008), four arrests for not having an operator's license within five years is classified as a felony (the same class of crime as murder). The law increases undocumented immigrants' risk of becoming felons as they are unable to obtain driver's licenses and are thus more likely to be arrested for not having a valid license while driving. Through this law, even if immigrants are able to escape ICE holds after being arrested for driving without a license four times, the four charges would effectively make them felons and likely result in their deportation being prioritized. By not giving undocumented immigrants a method of obtaining a driver's license, and by making driving without a license a felony, Georgia policies construct the very notions of criminal deviance that are often associated with "illegality."

Education restrictions and driving statutes point to how the Georgia legislature has made a concerted effort to restrict undocumented immigrants' mobility in numerous ways. In a literal, spatial sense, Georgia's policies restrict immigrants' mobility by criminalizing driving, which dramatically reduces a person's geographic range. More figuratively, and over the long term, Georgia's policies constrain immigrants' social mobility by restricting education and ultimately limiting their long-term economic opportunity. These efforts are part of Georgia's aggressive immigration enforcement regime.

Following examples set by California's Proposition 187 and Arizona's SB 1070, in 2011, the Georgia legislature passed HB 87. Georgia governor Nathan Deal campaigned on the promise of passing anti-immigrant legislation in Georgia, and he fulfilled his promise when he signed HB 87 into law. Before becoming governor, Deal had been a member of the U.S. House of Representatives, where he sat on the House Immigration Reform Caucus. The caucus pushed for legislation that "punished undocumented immigration," and promoted eliminating citizenship for children born in the United States to undocumented parents (Ku and Pervez 2010). Deal campaigned on immigration issues, and once elected, signed an anti-immigrant law and primed the legislature to continue passing anti-immigrant laws.

As described in the introduction, HB 87 requires that immigrants carry proof of their legal status at all times and authorizes local law enforcement to request proof of legal status from anyone suspected of being undocumented. When HB 87 passed, it also criminalized any form of assistance to undocumented immigrants, including transporting an undocumented person in a personal vehicle or providing any kind of nonemergency health service using public funds. Although the Eleventh Circuit Court of Appeals overturned the specific provisions regarding assisting undocumented immigrants, the rest of the law remains intact, including officers' authority to request proof of immigration status from anyone suspected of being undocumented. Just as with Arizona's SB 1070, the law has resulted in racially profiling Latinx immigrants, and as I later describe, it has created fear among some undocumented immigrants and confusion among some health providers. HB 87 also created the Immigration Enforcement and Review Board (IERB), which exists to ensure compliance with all immigration-related policies, as I describe in the following chapter.

While the purported rationale for HB 87 was to protect public funds and to punish undocumented immigrants, mirroring federal immigration laws of the past, the law conversely led to significant economic costs for Georgia. After Deal signed HB 87 into law, Latinx immigrants began leaving the state in such large numbers that the agricultural industry suffered a worker shortage and crops began rotting in fields. In the 2012 report from the Georgia Department of Agriculture, agricultural industry leaders who responded to a state survey about HB 87 and labor needs described a worker shortage directly related to Georgia's immigration law. As one respondent wrote, "Domestic American workers do not want to do farm labor—there was a shortage of Hispanic workers made worse by HB 87" (Georgia Department of Agriculture 2012, 102). To address the labor shortage, Governor Deal bused prisoners to farms to pick crops, but after less than half a day's work, the prisoners refused to continue working (Powell 2012). As a result of the labor shortage related to HB 87, Georgia's agricultural industry, the largest sector of the state economy, lost more than $1 billion in 2010 (Paluska 2011). Thus, targeting undocumented immigrants had significant financial costs for Georgia, but this has not discouraged policy makers from continuing to pass anti-immigrant legislation that I describe in the following chapter.

GOVERNING THROUGH CRIME TURNS TO GOVERNING THROUGH FEAR

As I have shown, immigration laws in the United States have historically responded to labor needs and been used as a way to maintain racial hierarchies. The multilevel immigrant policing regime affecting immigrants like Joaquín and inspiring CUCC protests in Marietta is an extension of U.S. immigration policy using race and health status to express immigrants' lack of belonging in the United States and to specifically deny immigrants' rights to publicly funded health services. Using crime and punishment as an additional context for asserting immigrants' lack of belonging, immigrant policing initiatives reinforce undocumented immigrants' racial otherness and directly impact their lives. As I continue demonstrating in the following chapters, immigrant policing regimes rooted in notions of immigrants' racial and criminal otherness have resulted in a fear-based governance strategy, where police officers and the threat of deportation are used to invoke terror among immigrant populations.

Invoking fear among immigrants is a deliberate political strategy, as Kris Kobach, vice chair of Donald Trump's "voter fraud commission" and drafter of Arizona's and Alabama's immigration enforcement laws, has indicated. Kobach has argued that immigration laws should encourage "self-deportation" (2008), presumably by making life as difficult as possible for immigrants in the United States. Despite these efforts, however, immigrants resist initiatives that encourage them to "self-deport," as CUCC protestors showed by demanding an end to HB 87, Neil Warren's policing practices, and 287(g) agreements.

In examining how policies like 287(g), Secure Communities, and HB 87 are part of a concerted effort to get immigrants to "self-deport," I argue that they use fear in a way that serves neoliberal aims. As anthropologist Aihwa Ong (2006) has shown, neoliberalism can be more than an economic philosophy: it can also be a biopolitical form of governmentality. Ong writes that neoliberalism focuses on individuals as "living resources that may be harnessed and managed by governing regimes" (2006, 6). Extending this argument, I assert that immigrant policing ultimately governs immigrants through fear to produce a new type of neoliberal citizen: one who hesitates to make demands on the state or seek social services and entitlements. This hyper-exploitative form of citizenship would not be possible, however, if it were not for the biopolitical processes of constructing immigrants as criminal, racial others. Producing a neoliberal citizen therefore serves political economic aims and also perpetuates the type of race-war construction Foucault (2003) describes that allows one population to go without specific resources and is justified by another group receiving those resources.

Constructing undocumented immigrants as criminal, racial others, and designing policies to make their lives so difficult that they "self-deport," reveals how "undocumentedness," or being undocumented, is a social status that may operate like other socially produced rationales for discrimination and inequality, such as race, class, and gender (Menjívar 2014). As a social status linked to inequality, undocumentedness continues to be a source of exclusion and vulnerability for nearly 11 million people living in the United States, all of whom are subjected to the kinds of insecurities associated with policing efforts. Moreover, immigrant policing efforts extend beyond individual immigrants to have much broader consequences that include altering immigrants' interpersonal relationships, health providers' professional practices, and the overall health safety net. In the following chapters, I describe the numerous health-related impacts of immigrant policing, but I first start with Georgia policy makers' rationales for passing laws like HB 87.

2 · INSIDE THE STATEHOUSE

Legislators' Perspectives on Georgia's Immigration Laws

On a sunny day in June, I got into Adelina's car and we drove from Atlanta to the more rural southern areas in Georgia. Over the course of a weekend, we visited communities outside of three towns: Tifton, Fitzgerald, and Warner Robbins. Adelina frequently drove across the state as part of GLAHR's grassroots organizing efforts to mobilize immigrants around ending aggressive immigration regimes. In many ways, this is what Adelina has been trained to do: she earned a sociology degree from the prestigious National Autonomous University of Mexico, and she had taught courses on social theory and methods. Before moving to the United States, Adelina had worked in rural communities in Mexico to inspire social and political organizing through popular education techniques—a type of social movement that makes education accessible to disenfranchised groups in order to effect social change. After she moved to Georgia, one of Adelina's first actions was traveling across the state collecting signatures for a petition to stop a law that banned undocumented immigrants from getting a driver's license.

Adelina and I drove down the highway passing vine-choked trees in a rental car, listening to Adelina's personal collection of social-justice-themed music. Occasionally, we would sing along. "¡El pueblo unido, jamás será vencido!" (The people united will never be defeated!)[1] Over the sound of a blowing air conditioner, I asked Adelina why she thought legislators started passing aggressive immigration enforcement laws in Georgia, including HB 87, the 2011 Arizona-style law that allowed police to arrest anyone suspected of being undocumented. "Because they are racist. They don't like immigrants," Adelina said.

When HB 87 was proposed, immigrant rights organizations such as GLAHR pointed to how it would encourage racial profiling, using Arizona's SB 1070 as an example. Other organizations, such as the American Civil Liberties Union (ACLU), argued some elements of the law were unconstitutional and ultimately sued the state once the law passed. Although proponents of the law indicated it would benefit Georgia's economy by targeting "criminal" immigrants who were "stealing" jobs and resources, by 2012 it had been well established that the law had harmed Georgia's economy by reducing the number of workers willing to engage in the state's largest industries, such as agriculture and hospitality. As Adelina observed, there was no evidence-driven basis for Georgia's most aggressive immigration law, but its nativist implications were clear.

Nativism—political positions and policies that favor native-born populations over immigrants—is woven through U.S. policy, as I described in the previous chapter. Anthropologist Leo Chavez argues nativist attitudes about Latinx populations center on constructing Latinx groups as a purported threat to the United States that will destroy the "American" way of life (2013, 2). At its core, what Chavez calls the "Latino threat narrative" hinges on protecting notions of whiteness, especially in Georgia, where lawmakers and anti-immigrant zealots worked together to pass a law that harmed the state's economy and, as I show in this chapter, expanded governmental bureaucracies.

"You know we had a Latino vote for [HB 87]?" Adelina asked me, incredulously, as we continued our drive south. "David Casas *Sí, 'manito.* He voted for it and he is Latino. We call him 'David Homes.'" By anglicizing his name, Adelina hinted at the racial politics behind HB 87 and other immigration laws. Laws like HB 87 were designed to protect whiteness, and it made little sense for someone that white legislators might consider nonwhite to support such a policy.

In each town we stopped, Adelina met with local community members in churches to share information about 287(g), Secure Communities, and HB 87. This process was part of her grassroots organizing strategy based on a popular education approach. During these meetings, community members shared stories about being stopped by police, getting arrested, and needing advice. In one town, Beta, a farmworker in her late twenties from Mexico, sat with her two small children worrying about having been arrested several weeks earlier.

"They stopped me because they said my [tail]light was out, but I *always* check it. I *always* check my lights and I know it was okay. I was in jail for three days and I have this fine. . . . I have to go to court." Beta looked at Adelina, then over to her children, and back to Adelina. "What do I do?"

Adelina (see figure 1) photographed Beta's documents with her phone. "Give me your phone number and I'll take this back to the office and see what I can find out." She then redirected her attention to the three others in the room. "This is why we have to organize—these types of injustices! We can help you organize and confront local police and demand that they stop pulling people over just because they are Latino." In one of the most rural areas of the state, the impacts of immigrant policing regimes could not be clearer: HB 87 emboldened rural police to racially profile drivers like Beta; once arrested, Beta could be deported, leaving behind her children and leaving the crops she picked for a living to rot in

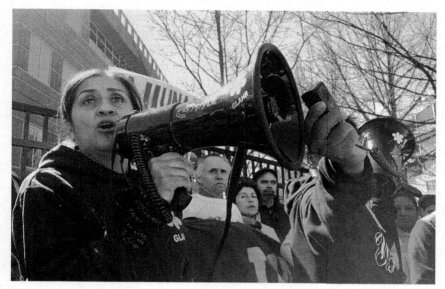

FIGURE 1. Adelina holding a megaphone at a rally. (Photo by Laura Emiko Soltis.)

the Georgia sun. In an effort to organize the meeting attendees, Adelina suggested marches and issuing demands to the police. Her passionate and compelling plea inspired nods in the room, but some expressed discomfort with the idea of exposing themselves to local police, asking why Adelina could not just deal with the police herself. "Because I don't live here," Adelina answered. "I live in Atlanta. You all are the ones that live here and face this every day."

In every town we visited, we heard stories like Beta's at gatherings of four to twenty people. Two towns had few attendees, which Adelina suspected was the result of poor communication between points of contact and community members. "The pastor [at the church where we met community members] reminds people the meeting is happening so they come—he says he did it, but I think he forgot." After our final stop in the two-day trip and during our drive back to Atlanta, Adelina reflected on stories she heard during our visits to the three towns.

"These stories are so typical—'I got stopped for no seatbelt,' or 'I got stopped for a broken taillight,' or they just stop people for no reason at all. It's destroying our community," Adelina said staring at the road, occasionally interjecting with comments about other drivers' recklessness. "We have to fight these anti-immigrant laws. *Pinche cabrón* [fucking asshole]! You see that? No turn signal [from the driver of a car that nearly hit us]." Stories like Beta's, which were reminiscent of Esme and Alvaro's, were similar to other narratives of immigrant policing I heard while living in Atlanta, demonstrating how localized immigration enforcement often operated through 287(g), Secure Communities, and HB 87.

In this chapter, I examine Georgia policy makers' perspectives on immigrant policing efforts that affected Beta, Esme and Alvaro, and countless other immigrants in Georgia. I draw from interviews with legislators, conversations with lobbyists, and participant observation experiences in the state capitol and at Immigration Enforcement and Review Board (IERB) meetings to assess legislators' aims in passing HB 87 and other immigration laws that advance localized immigration enforcement agendas. I examine the relationship between state legislators and one anti-immigrant organization leader, Donald Allen (DA) King, and describe the challenges anthropologists can have when trying to study governmental power. As I show in this chapter, legislators' support of laws like HB 87 can be understood through Foucault's notion of race-war logics (2003) that speaks to racial anxieties about demographic changes in Georgia and in Atlanta especially. Because undocumented immigration is a politically expedient topic, legislators' support for immigration laws like HB 87 can be understood as what sociologists Nikolas Rose and Carlos Novas call "citizenship projects" (2007), which encompass ways in which policy makers act on certain groups of people.

THE GEORGIA CAPITOL

The layered immigration enforcement regime in Georgia reflects the overall layered U.S. system of government that includes the national federal government and individual state governments. As the capital of Georgia, Atlanta is home to the state legislature, which I frequented during my fieldwork. Like the federal government, Georgia's legislature is divided into a House and Senate, and bills proposed in one chamber of the legislature must pass the other in order to become law. The origin of a bill is marked in its name (Senate Bill, or SB, versus House Bill, or HB), and both chambers of the legislature proposed immigration bills during my fieldwork. In the 2013 Georgia legislative session, I frequented the state capitol to meet with legislators, lobbyists, and activists, and I attempted to get information about specific immigration-related bills.

The interior of the Georgia capitol looks like a blend of U.S. federal government buildings and how I imagine a local sheriff's office from the early 1900s looked in a small Georgia town. White marble floors, Roman columns, and stone balustrades bounce noise across the open spaces and against deep-brown wooden doors with transoms and Main Street–style lampposts with globe casings that cast dull glows from incandescent bulbs (see figure 2). The capitol was frequently hectic when the state legislature, known as the General Assembly, met, but guards often recognized repeated visitors, including me on a day I went to look for Matt Ramsey, the Republican co-sponsor of HB 87.

In many ways, politics in Georgia mirror federal politics: there are two political parties (Democrats and Republicans) that adhere to differing ideological platforms. As seen among members in the U.S. Congress and in Republican presi-

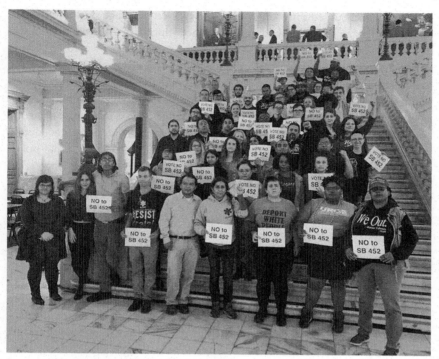

FIGURE 2. Inside Georgia's capitol, GLAHRiadores hold up signs to oppose SB 452, which was debated in the 2017–2018 legislative session. (Photo by GLAHR.)

dent Donald Trump, Republicans in Georgia are more likely to support aggressive immigration regimes than Democrats. Among lobbyists I met in Georgia, Matt Ramsey was considered to be synonymous with immigration enforcement laws, and as a member of the Georgia House of Representatives, he co-sponsored HB 87. I repeatedly tried to schedule interviews with Matt Ramsey, and his assistant typically found reasons why he could not meet with me—often legislative meetings or attending his son's baseball games.

One day, after receiving several excuses for why Ramsey could not meet to discuss immigration with me, I told his assistant I specifically wanted to discuss HB 87. I noted that Democrats had been willing to conduct an interview, but Republicans, including those who supported immigration laws, had refused. "I'm trying to reach out to everyone I can about HB 87 and I'd really like to talk to Mr. Ramsey since he's the most knowledgeable," I explained. I then argued it would be unfair to capture *only* Democrats' perspectives, and Ramsey's assistant ultimately agreed. "Oh, that's very true," she exclaimed, "and we certainly don't want only their voices heard!" We eventually scheduled a meeting, but Ramsey's assistant warned, "It's nothing definite, but I'll see what I can do. Write down your number and I'll let him know you stopped by—we certainly want both sides to be heard!"

The day I scheduled a meeting with Ramsey, I left his office suite and went to meet with Jim[2], a lobbyist I had gotten to know during my time in Atlanta. He had been helpful in providing me a list of legislators he knew would talk to me and had given me background information about how HB 87 passed. According to Jim, HB 87 passed as an accident because other legislation related to taxes and health insurance failed to materialize in a passable bill. Although Republicans campaigned on HB 87, Jim claimed they never intended to pass it because of strong opposition from agricultural leaders; but once other bills failed, they needed to pass legislation to appear productive to voters. He further suggested that political maneuvering between the bill's sponsors, Matt Ramsey and Chip Rogers, led other Republicans to vote for the bill. "Matt Ramsey is a powerful figure. . . . He controls a lot of the party's lines on issues," Jim explained.

Because Ramsey was a co-sponsor of HB 87 and central Republican leader, I had hoped to meet and speak with him and get his perspective on the law and the impetus for it. Speaking to his assistant seemed promising. When I met up with Jim the day I saw Ramsey's assistant, he immediately asked if I had talked to Ramsey. I told him no. He asked who else I intended on speaking with, and I told him I would talk to anyone who had anything to do with HB 87, to which Jim replied by laughing at me. "Good luck!" A smile stretched across his face. "Republicans aren't going to speak to *anyone* about that. . . . They're not going to talk about this; party leadership won't let it happen." Jim was right. On Thursday afternoon of that week I received a phone call from Ramsey's assistant informing me that the Friday meeting we had scheduled would not work for him and that a meeting while the General Assembly was in session was unlikely to happen.

The obstruction I experienced in trying to meet Matt Ramsey mirrored other ways Georgia Republicans ignored my efforts to speak to them. Republican legislators either rejected interview invitations, never responded to emails and phone calls, or had assistants who continually informed me of their inability to meet with me due to busy schedules while assuring me I was not being ignored. As one assistant insisted about another Republican supporter of HB 87: "He's got a law practice, a wife, plays baseball, and has a little one at home, so he's not ignoring you, he's just busy." Somehow, though, legislators who opposed HB 87 and had similar obligations still found time to meet with me.

Despite never meeting with Republican legislators, I was able to interview Democrats who were vocally against HB 87. I had hoped to speak with supporters of HB 87 and those who opposed the law to get a robust understanding of the politics informing state-level immigration laws. This effort effectively categorized interviewees into one political party or another, as co-sponsors and public supporters of HB 87 were all Republicans, and the vocal opposition to the law were all Democrats. One of the most vocal Democrats, House Minority Leader Stacey Abrams, was most willing to share a perspective about immigration laws in Georgia and immigrant policing.

Abrams has been described as a political "up and comer" among Atlanta progressives. She is the first woman to lead a political party in the Georgia General Assembly and the first African American to lead in the Georgia House (Friends of Stacey Y. Abrams 2014). She is trained in sociology and public affairs and holds a law degree from Yale. She continues to rise to national prominence, and in 2017 she entered Georgia's race for governor and became the first woman to win a gubernatorial primary in Georgia. As House minority leader, she set the political discourse for the Democrats in the Georgia House of Representatives, making her an ideal interviewee to provide insight about legislators' opinions from her own party. When I asked her about HB 87, Abrams contextualized Georgia as a state with a deep history of racial and class-based divisions, further subdivided by urban and rural settings that have strong economies and require immigrant labor.

> You have a deep agricultural history, which has led to the need for immigrant labor, but there's always been a little bit of hostility about it because immigrant labor basically dispossessed sharecropper labor.[3] We've got this complicated history of race and class that has always been part of the state, and then you add to that the fact that if you're in the north the immigrant labor is used for chicken processing, and if you're in towns or in tourist areas it's used for restaurants. So in economic boom times, things are fine because you have this mutual coexistence because [immigrants and nonimmigrants are not] fighting over anything.

As Abrams indicated, immigrants in Georgia have worked in agricultural, textile, and poultry industries in rural parts of the state. When immigrants like Joaquín started moving to the Atlanta area as part of the construction boom related to the 1996 Olympic Games, the number of immigrants in Atlanta and its surrounding suburbs increased. As I explained in the previous chapter, the suburban settlement pattern and the rapidly growing Latinx population resulted in predominantly white legislators, local government officials, and suburban residents enacting a series of laws and ordinances to restrict Latinx immigrants' access to housing, education, health services, and transportation (Browne and Odem 2012). These ordinances are built on the foundation of Jim Crow policies that historically reinforced racial segregation of blacks and whites in the U.S. South, resulting in a new set of "Juan Crow" laws targeting Latinx groups (Browne and Odem 2012).

Further tying together race, labor, rural and urban divides, and immigration, Abrams explained how the rise of anti-immigrant sentiment and immigration laws passing the state legislature were connected to Georgia's economic decline, bad policies, and immigrant scapegoating rooted in a history of racial discrimination: "The genesis of this antagonism isn't anything new or illustrative of some zeitgeist taking over the state. It really is reflective of the cycles of history, which are that when you have lack of anything or [face some type of] a challenge, you always blame the thing that doesn't look like you, and to the extent that you can create an alien presence and dehumanize it then that becomes much more aggressive." Linking processes of dehumanization to economic concerns, Abrams added: "You add all that together with the fact that north Georgia in 2010 faced a dramatic economic decline, and that was the hub for a lot of the economic success for the state." She pointed to a map of Georgia hanging on her wall. "North Georgia is about one-third of the map. They were producing all of the couches and carpets and all of the furniture and everything that was going into the housing boom that was fueling Georgia . . . and they were hiring a lot of undocumented persons to do the work. When it all collapsed," she continued, referring to the national housing market collapse, "you suddenly had to explain why we had all these Latinos, and to a lesser extent Asians, but mostly Latinos, living in these communities that were predominantly white and never really had to coexist peacefully with other communities." As Abrams noted, the genesis of laws like HB 87 stemmed from an economic decline that made use of available labor from immigrants like Joaquín, but when the economy worsened, the demographic changes in areas that accompanied labor transformations resulted in heightened anti-immigrant sentiments. "Suddenly [elected officials] had to explain why there were no jobs available to all the people who elected [them]," she added. "So despite having *every* major corporation saying that [HB 87] is a bad idea, despite having *every* national figure we could muster talk about why this is terrible . . . the political power center had to explain why their economy was collapsing, and it was either the Republicans' fault or immigrants' fault. They picked the immigrants."

Much like national immigration policy throughout U.S. history, Georgia's immigration policies included racial anxieties and concerns that immigrants might use social services. Economic scapegoating of immigrants further coincided with critiques of the federal government's alleged inability to control costs of entitlement programs and failure to appropriately respond to immigration concerns. "The articulated reason was cost," Abrams explained, "and [Republicans claimed] we had to act because the federal government didn't." Other legislators I spoke to also mentioned the failure of the federal government to act, and Abrams, like others, felt this was a reasonable argument. "I think [the federal government issue] might be legitimate except that state laws have never served to actually stop or thwart unlawful activity when it comes to immigration."[4] Similarly, immigration laws that passed in other states largely drew from a rhetoric of federal government failure to justify state legislation focusing on immigrants (Lacey and Rodriguez 2011). Despite justifying laws like HB 87 as economically necessary and required at a state level because of federal inaction, in some locations, like Georgia, business leaders have argued that immigration laws have contributed to economic hardships.

In June 2011, at a meeting in downtown Atlanta titled "Forging Consensus," a group of political conservatives met to discuss national immigration reform in a

Georgia context. The event featured Alberto Gonzales, the U.S. attorney general during the George W. Bush administration, and talks from local academics, attorneys, chamber of commerce representatives, law enforcement agents, agricultural industry representatives, and politicians, who described the economic importance of immigrants in Georgia. John King, chief of police for Doraville, an Atlanta suburb with a large immigrant population, spoke about the harm of aggressive immigration enforcement, noting that it eroded trust among local immigrants. "[Section 287(g)] has complicated my relationship with my community and has made it difficult for me to protect the community," King asserted. Further, some of the speakers, including a representative from the Georgia Restaurant Association and the mayor of the small agricultural town Uvalda, discussed the negative economic impacts of HB 87, arguing that it resulted in fewer immigrant workers to fill service economy and agricultural jobs (Georgia Restaurant Association, n.d.; Trevizo 2012). The dialogue at the "Forging Consensus" meeting emphasized that Latinx workers who picked Georgia's crops and worked in the back of the local restaurants provided substantive economic benefits to the state, and it further revealed that political conservatives were well aware of negative impacts of immigrant policing regimes.

When I asked Abrams if Georgia legislators would change HB 87 because of data indicating its economic and social costs, she argued that changing the law would be politically difficult: "There is no political will to fix it because you have to admit out loud that it was a mistake." She continued, adding that ultimately the law would operate with some degree of inaction by the board designated to oversee the law, the IERB. "Let's take the IERB as an example," Abrams said, noting the IERB's function to ensure compliance with HB 87. "The largest noncompliant sector is agriculture and it's for a reason. What we've done is essentially nullify our own laws through our agency inaction. . . . A great deal of the law was nullified by [a court] decision, then more of it was nullified simply by inaction." The result, Abrams explained, would be an unenforceable law. "Ultimately what we will have is [a] really, really awful law on the books but very little enforcement, which I think is the intent. You know, you got the bang for the buck which is in an election year, you got to say that you hated immigrants but in reality hurt the economy, and now will do very little to actually enforce it." To Abrams, then, keeping HB 87 in place but not enforcing elements that were inconvenient for certain industries was precisely what the legislature wanted to do.

As I noted earlier, HB 87 created the IERB, which is staffed by appointees from the governor and the lieutenant governor. The appointees are charged with ensuring broad compliance with HB 87, but in some situations, the IERB ignored HB 87 requirements. Despite the IERB not enforcing all aspects of the law, HB 87 and other immigrant policing efforts nevertheless had numerous consequences on immigrants, health professionals, and the entire medical system, as I show throughout this book. Moreover, anti-immigrant activists like Cobb County local DA King routinely attended IERB meetings and argued for board members to be aggressive in their compliance efforts. As Abrams noted, members of anti-immigrant groups like those that intimidated CUCC members in Marietta would never relent in their complaints: "We lost $3 billion [in agricultural revenue]. . . . But the zeal, the zealotry that [some] bring to this issue will not go away because there's the political dynamic which says this is a good way to get elected and then there's just the true xenophobia that says that these people are somehow evil and unworthy and that doesn't disappear."

TRACING POLICIES TO ANTI-IMMIGRANT ACTIVISTS AND UNDERSTANDING THE CONSEQUENCES

Like Abrams, other legislators also discussed xenophobia and racism as part of immigrant policing efforts, pointing not just to state legislation but also to county ordinances restricting undocumented immigrants from certain types of housing. As one legislator said to me, "Cherokee County back in 1999 tried to pass a law focusing on rentals. They wanted to not allow rental units to people without documents." The same legislator commented on DA King's influence with some state lawmakers, noting that his organization was one of the largest anti-immigrant groups in the state. King's organization routinely held demonstrations and rallies to show its opposition to undocumented immigrants living in Georgia. His organization's website features content espousing explicitly anti-"illegal" immigrant messages and claiming credit for two of Georgia's immigration laws, including HB 87. The site also features lists of individuals and organizations allegedly "encouraging, assisting, and profiting from illegal immigration," which includes names of local NGO officials and activists, like Rich—the man whose dog was murdered and placed on his doorstep. Among the organizations listed are international nonprofits such as the Anti-Defamation League, which combats anti-Semitism and bigotry, and the Ford Foundation, which advances a number of causes related to human welfare.

Legislators, lobbyists, and activists often commented on King's political ties to Republican lawmakers in Georgia. According to one legislator I interviewed, DA King was a "sidekick" to Republican lawmaker and HB 87 co-sponsor, Representative Chip Rogers. Jim explained that Chip Rogers and other Republican legislators used King as a mouthpiece to reach a set of conservative voters connected to anti-immigrant and conservative organizations. "He's really radical, and he's a gatekeeper to a bunch of groups, so they allowed him to voice ideas for legislation. He's the official representative of FAIR [Federation for American Immigration Reform—a conservative anti-undocumented immigrant organization] through his organization." In many ways, King and Georgia Republican lawmakers used one another: legislators reached a radical group of political conservatives through King, and King got to see his group's radical views represented in the state-house and reflected in legislation like HB 87.

Anti-immigrant legislation like HB 87 may appease immigration opponents like DA King, but it ultimately harms states like Georgia. As I have already indicated, HB 87 had negative financial consequences on Georgia's agricultural and restaurant industries, but the law also created a professional licensing problem that plagued Georgia officials and resulted in massive governmental inefficiencies.

In the United States, some occupations require licensure to legally practice the profession. HB 87 required anyone with a professional license, such as a medical, nursing, or even a cosmetology license, to prove their citizenship when renewing their licensure. This placed a burden on state workers to assess and validate professionals' citizenship status, resulting in what some lawmakers and lobbyists referred to as "a bureaucratic nightmare" for the state. As one legislator noted: "That section [of HB 87] that says that if you're licensed in the state of Georgia, every time that you renew, you have to show your citizenship . . . the Secretary of State came out swinging saying that they don't have the budget or the manpower to review all of the nurses, the doctors, the cosmetologists." With too few staff to comply with a process created as a result of HB 87, the secretary of state's office, which handles basic administrative tasks, was delayed in approving professional license renewals. As I describe in chapter 5, this resulted in some U.S. citizen workers, including health workers, risking their legal ability to practice their profession as the approval time took as much as three times longer than normal. "Everyone that has to have a renewal of the license was backlogged; nurses were usually going 20 days and this is going to take about three months for them," the legislator added.

Anti-immigrant groups and anti-immigrant protestors like DA King may have played a role in crafting laws like HB 87, but such laws ultimately do more harm than good. In addition to the deleterious consequences for Georgia's economy, HB 87 ultimately created a mess for the state government and anyone working in a field with a professional license. This particular immigrant policing effort, then, made government processes more cumbersome and burdened a large section of Georgia's professional workforce. The professional licensing renewal problems resulting from HB 87 were so significant that they required subsequent legislation, which was discussed at IERB meetings.

SHROUDED IN SECRECY: STUDYING THE STATE AND ITS INSTRUMENTS

When HB 87 established the IERB, it gave the governor and the lieutenant governor the authority to appoint the board's members and any future members who are needed to fill vacancies due to any board member's resignation. The IERB holds ad hoc public meetings and reviews complaints that allege noncompliance with HB 87. Anyone can file a complaint, and complaints can include assertions about how municipalities, counties, or other local governments violate specific provisions related to HB 87. For example, if a local municipality were to decide it would provide free preventive health care at a local public clinic to all residents regardless of citizenship, it would specifically violate a provision in HB 87 that criminalizes using public funds to provide services to undocumented immigrants. Through creating the IERB to ensure compliance with HB 87, HB 87 added a layer of surveilling immigrants on top of the surveillance efforts associated with granting local police discretion to stop immigrants on the basis of their suspected immigration status. Local police surveil immigrants, and the IERB surveils local governments and their associated agencies.

The IERB has no legislative history or documented public debate about its creation, and it was a surprise addition to HB 87 (Kuck 2011). It serves to hear complaints about local governments' alleged violations of HB 87, investigate them, and take whatever action the board deems appropriate. It is empowered to make its own rules, subpoena documents, and place witnesses under oath for testimony regarding alleged violations of HB 87. The board has a wide enforcement purview that includes, for example, ensuring public agencies and employees properly enforce the use of E-Verify—an electronic system to check eligibility to work in the United States by comparing data an employer enters with federal records. Further, the IERB is charged with ensuring that local governments comply with state policies that prohibit "sanctuary" cities or counties—which are, in the broadest sense, local governments that limit cooperation with immigration enforcement authorities. Georgia officially banned sanctuary cities in 2010 and in 2016 passed legislation (Senate Bill 269) requiring governments to cooperate with immigration officials in order to receive state funding. The IERB also monitors local governments' use of the Systematic Alien Verification for Entitlements (SAVE) system—a program verifying immigration status for public benefit applications, such as enrolling in the Supplemental Nutritional Assistance Program (SNAP), the U.S. program aimed at alleviating hunger among low-income populations. More alarming than what the IERB does, however, is who composes the board and the IERB's relationship to DA King. In 2018, the Southern Poverty Law Center (2018) asserted that the IERB effectively served as King's "personal public investigative agency," noting King's ties to white nationalists and Georgia legislators.

While conducting the fieldwork that resulted in this book, I attended four public meetings of the IERB. King was present for three meetings and filed complaints that were discussed in all of them. King was responsible for a series of complaints brought against Georgia's Department of Audits (DoA), Department of Community Affairs (DCA), and other state agencies and local municipalities, alleging one municipality was a sanctuary city for undocumented immigrants and that DCA and DoA failed to prohibit undocumented immigrants from receiving

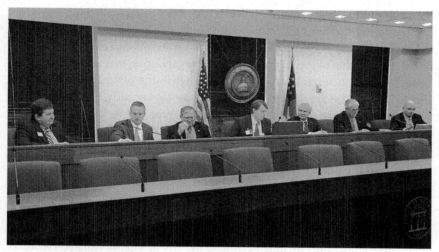

FIGURE 3. Members of the IERB. (Photo by Nolan Kline.)

state benefits. King alleged these state agencies and municipalities violated HB 87, and urged the IERB to take action.

The IERB met quarterly, and meetings were usually announced with little advance notice and were not widely broadcasted even though they were open to the public. Few, if any, members of the public attended other than journalists. Through my affiliation with the Georgia Immigrant and Refugee Rights Coalition (GIRRC), I learned about IERB meetings, which were held in a legislative office building across the street from the capitol. The legislative office buildings housed spaces for legislators, including Stacey Abrams, and meeting rooms used for events such as the ACLU's "By the People" legislative days, at which the ACLU provided suggestions for how constituents could best communicate their concerns to legislators. The board consists of seven members, all of whom had some affiliation with the Georgia Republican Party during my fieldwork. When I attended meetings (see figure 3), the board members included attorney Ben Vinson; former journalist Phil Kent; government relations consultant and Georgia Department of Veterans Service board member Shawn Hanley; mayor of Dallas, Georgia, Boyd Austin; Coweta County sheriff Mike Yeager; attorney Robert Mumford; and Colquitt County commissioner Terry Clark. Republican state senator (then just a state senate hopeful) John Kennedy replaced Robert Mumford in one of the final meetings I attended and was appointed by the governor and the lieutenant governor.

One of the IERB members, Phil Kent, was a particularly controversial choice for the board. One legislator I interviewed claimed Kent had connections to hate groups and anti-immigrant organizations, saying, "Oh, he's evil." After Kent was appointed to the IERB, the Southern Poverty Law Center claimed Kent was a

"Hate Group Leader," citing his role as a member of a radical anti-immigration organization, Americans for Immigration Control, which is perhaps most notable for advocating an end to certain types of birthright citizenship, and Kent's board membership of ProEnglish: a national organization that actively promotes English-only policies and strives to make English the official language of the United States (Beirich and Southern Poverty Law Center 2011). Kent's ties to anti-immigrant organizations is alarming given his official role on the IERB and authority to administer sanctions to agencies and municipalities deemed noncompliant with HB 87. Similarly, Kent and other board members have questionable connections to King. Kent and other IERB members were often friendly with King, and Kent in particular displayed a sense of admiration for King by pushing for him to be able to address the IERB and ardently siding with his positions during meetings.

The IERB meetings I attended all revolved around complaints that King had filed. These complaints included claiming the city of Vidalia violated Georgia's sanctuary city policy and that the DCA, DoA, and hundreds of other state agencies were not compliant with SAVE system requirements put in place by HB 87. In several meetings King referred to himself in ways that suggested closeness with legislators, once describing what he saw to be his hand in drafting HB 87: "In 2009 we altered Georgia code—and I say 'we' because I'm regarded as furniture around here—to ensure applicants for entitlements be checked against the SAVE program for eligibility." The SAVE program was one of King's frequent talking points, and he argued that lack of compliance with SAVE cost taxpayers money through granting undocumented immigrants benefits. King seemed to make reporting compliance errors a personal hobby, if not a full-time job, for himself (see figure 4).

At one meeting, King presented his arguments against agencies not complying with HB 87 and sought action from the IERB (Redmon 2012). He asserted that under HB 87, all government agencies were required to file reports with DCA and DoA regarding their use of SAVE and E-Verify systems. King argued that since agencies were not submitting their reports, DCA and DoA were failing to comply with HB 87. This assertion ultimately led the IERB, at the urging of Phil Kent, to conduct an investigation of the DCA and DoA to assess whether the numerous entities under their purview were using the SAVE system when assessing benefit eligibility for applicants and the E-Verify system when hiring employees. In a meeting where DCA and DoA representatives had to respond to the allegations against them, DCA commissioner Mike Beatty and DoA director Carol Schwinne appeared before the IERB and responded to King's complaints and the IERB's concerns. Beatty explained that the alleged noncompliance was due to not all agencies being aware of the requirements, and he appeared to try not to upset King.

"Being a former legislator, I appreciate abiding by the law, and I appreciate the enthusiasm of people like DA King," Beatty cautiously began one statement at a

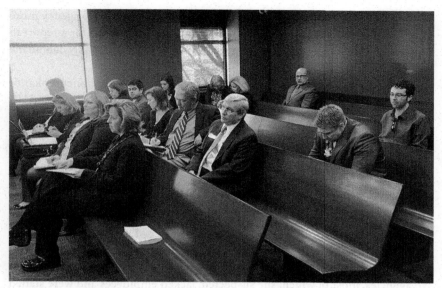

FIGURE 4. DA King staring at the photographer, Roberto Gutierrez, during an IERB meeting, where King was seated in the last row.

meeting. In that statement, Beatty claimed that although not all DCA institutions were complying with the requirements to check entitlement applications against SAVE, he offered that he would work with the governor to ensure all agencies complied by the end of the year and educate agencies, explaining it was "a culture change" since HB 87 passed. "If we messed it up, we messed up trying to do what was right," Beatty pleaded. "We'll do what we can to make sure everyone complies with this. I think there are great people in this state and, Lord, we just have to get the information out! We want to make sure people are using SAVE the right way for those public benefits."

In an attempt to explain potential problems with getting all entities compliant, IERB member Boyd Austin noted that some government agencies, including small towns, lacked internet capability, so 100 percent compliance might take time. King, who had been standing during Beatty's presentation, interrupted Austin and asked to be recognized to speak. "I enjoyed Mike's presentation about his office not being in compliance with the law, but the size of the city is not relevant," he asserted. IERB member Ben Vinson, nodding to King, said he appreciated King's comments, and Kent charged that the board needed to act. "We need to make an example out of agencies not complying with the law!" he exclaimed. Austin, in a more reasonable approach to understanding noncompliance claims, suggested that there was more to the situation. "I don't think it's as willful as people think it is," Austin interjected, stating that agencies and municipalities are not likely to be willingly noncompliant with the law. "But we don't know that!" Kent retorted.

Ultimately the board agreed to investigate the DCA, allowed the agency more time to understand who complied and who did not, and waited for a report to explain the situation. This decision annoyed King, who scoffed loudly behind me in the hearing room.

The DoA had a less difficult time than DCA responding to noncompliance charges. In addressing the complaint against her agency, Schwinne explained HB 87 required her department to develop a website that explained all governments should notify her office about contracts to ensure contractors were using E-Verify. Since "governments" are defined as any entity receiving public funding of any kind, her office expected to hear from a very large number of agencies. When the deadline to deliver this information arrived, there were 1,170 noncompliant government agencies, prompting her office to send letters requesting information. The information request DoA sent was to assess whether reporting information was needed; any agency without paid staff would not need to report, so her office felt the request for information was an appropriate way to determine who should and should not be reporting. Schwinne's office lacked responses from 570 agencies, most of which, she suspected, lacked employees and were staffed by volunteers, so they were exempt from providing information the DoA requested. Through responding to questions from the IERB members, Schwinne explained that the list of government agencies required to provide information can change every year since it includes school boards, development authorities, and other potentially changing organizations that do not have employees but can be staffed by volunteers, and that her office was attempting to determine how to manage the challenges associated with these circumstances. After Schwinne's explanation of alleged violations, Vinson invited King to respond to Schwinne and the DoA.

Rather than rebutting Schwinne's points in his response to the DoA, King refocused on DCA and Beatty, especially. "The spirit of the law was to protect jobs," King began. He claimed to have spent his own money traveling across the state to investigate whether county commissioners were aware of HB 87's requirements. Ending his tirade, he announced: "I'll be filing papers with the Attorney General tomorrow to pursue civil action against DCA since the board is not taking action." Vinson thanked King and asked Beatty about DCA's compliance efforts, and Beatty explained DCA was "working on it." Kent, watching King, who stood in the back, quickly accused DCA of failing to comply with HB 87. "But you really aren't in compliance!" he exclaimed. Beatty promptly asked for assistance from someone accompanying him, who stood and firmly rebutted Kent's accusation. "We're in compliance with HB 87 and with E-Verify, so to say we're not is not correct." Ultimately the board agreed to allow DCA more time to address the complaint King brought and did not settle the DoA affair. By the following meeting, which occurred three months later, King had withdrawn his complaint against DoA but continued his complaint against the DCA.

At the next meeting, a DCA division director, John Turner, addressed the board about King's complaint, arguing that DCA had made changes to address the complaint against the agency. Turner's explanation was not satisfactory to King, however, who railed against DCA and state agencies for not following HB 87. In a dramatic gesture, King called for Beatty's resignation, claiming that someone aware of laws and not needing to be coerced into compliance through the threat of a complaint should be running DCA. He then expressed surprise that the board had not used its authority to place people under oath and make them testify about his complaints. After King's tirade, Kent demanded an evidentiary hearing, but no one was entirely clear on what issue. In front of me, two reporters looked to each other trying to understand what was happening. "Are you following any of this?" one asked. "No," another responded, laughing. All that was clear was that King was angry, Kent was motivated by King's anger, and the board was moving to take some type of action against DCA.

Ultimately the board agreed to have a hearing, and Kent asserted it must be done expeditiously. When the board agreed to have a hearing thirty to forty-five days after the meeting, Kent invited King to address the board, adding that perhaps legislators who may need to alter HB 87 attend the hearing. King offered to recommend to the board which legislators should attend and would be amenable to changing immigration laws. He specifically added that the language needed to be altered in a piece of legislation so that entities that do not provide a public benefit are clearly required to file a report making that fact clear. King again asserted that the DCA commissioner should resign, and volunteered to be hired for the job because he claimed he already did it for free. Kent responded by saying he would like to hear more legislation recommendations, and King said he would provide more recommendations later. Turner, seemingly frustrated and incredulous about what was unfolding, explained that the DCA was not a regulatory agency, and that DCA could only send a notice to entities informing them of their need to report under the law.

"DCA wants to be in compliance but has no means by which the agency can require public entities in Georgia to register and report their public benefits programs," he asserted. Despite this explanation, no changes were made, and the board adjourned for another three months. In short, the DCA was being held accountable for something the agency leaders felt it had either satisfied or could not accomplish, all under the guise of being "tough on immigration." This type of bureaucratic performance made little sense to reporters or to me, and I became increasingly interested in why some board members found King to be credible.

At the March 2013 IERB meeting, connections between King and the IERB members began to crystallize. Before the meeting began, I made my way through security and into the elevator. As I exited the elevator, Kent approached King, who was standing with two other people that eventually accompanied him into the meeting. Kent smiled, and called to King. "Hey, I've seen you on TV!" Kent exclaimed, suggesting King had celebrity status. King laughed and the two of them began talking with three other people accompanying King before making their way into the hearing room. During the IERB meeting, King withdrew his complaint against DCA, claiming the current law would not allow for additional sanctions. He then requested the board focus on a complaint he filed eight months prior, claiming the board had not fulfilled its obligation to respond to complaints in sixty days. Vinson responded by explaining the IERB was staffed by unpaid volunteers (since its creation did not accompany funds for staff) and was only required to review complaints internally within sixty days and did not have to take action within sixty days. Kent pressed King's point, and Vinson, seemingly annoyed, explained the challenges in addressing the complaint, which listed hundreds of agencies allegedly not complying with HB 87. "A shotgun complaint against 600 entities proves problematic for the board; there is no staff, and our budget allows money for staff but should be used for court reporters and subpoenas." Kent responded by insisting the board act. "These are entities that refuse to report to the Department of Community Affairs and we should choose a few, five-ten, to go after and make an example to show this board has some real teeth in enforcing the law!"

One of the women accompanying King, Kay Godwin, a leader of a local conservative political organization, stood up during the meeting and demanded the board take some type of action. Following Godwin, King asserted the board was failing to do anything to change the current situation and said he was stunned by the attitude of the chair saying the IERB would not investigate 600 agencies. King argued that the board was not operating in the spirit of the law and that it was burdening citizens like himself with an unnecessary task in ensuring it had credible and specific complaints. "If the action is to make the citizen who is aware of the violators find the time and money to itemize every separate written complaint," King angrily stated, "I don't believe that is in the spirit or intent of the law."

IERB member Hanley directly responded to King. "It's just . . . you can or you can't—the reality is that there are 600. We're the investigators—we're it, that's just the reality. . . . Nobody is more incensed about the degree of lawbreaking across this country and across this state when it comes to illegal immigration," Hanley claimed, seeming to express sympathy with King's frustration. "It sickens me to a high degree that we go through this every day on our roads and everything else," he added. It was unclear to me what sickened Hanley, exactly. Was he "sickened" that there were immigrants driving on local roadways, or that they dared to live in areas where he might see them? He continued, and explained that he was willing to work with King. "But DA, you have to take a look at what we're doing," he said. "We're doing the best we can, the chairman is doing the best he can—unfortunately there is a procedural issue we have to take care of. We want to make sure this board—we want to go after every single agency we can—that's the issue." Further suggesting the practical problems of examining how compliant agencies were with HB 87, Hanley added: "We're not going to go bouncing around to 600 agencies because it's not going to be a very good investigation, sorry, but it's not. I'd appreciate you to rethink it and say 'how can I get the most out of the board? How can I drill down and get 10?' This is an opportunity for you to work with us."

With Hanley's direction, the conversation refocused on the need for due process and the requirement of specificity in complaints rather than large blanket accusations claiming hundreds or thousands of agencies are not compliant with HB 87. After tense dialogue between King and various board members, Godwin stood up and accused the board of failing to address existing laws. "I don't understand why we're passing laws if we're not going to hold people accountable for what they do!" Godwin exclaimed. "If we are allowing mass groups of people to just simply ignore the law, why are we making them in the first place? This is ridiculous, I mean we're supposed to be a state of laws, and we're supposed to obey them however you have to obey them!" Becoming increasingly animated, Godwin suggested the board's request for a reasonable number of agencies to investigate was unnecessary. "I can't imagine singling out one or two; I mean either you investigate every one of them and prove them right or wrong or just forget it! Let's just don't even have law! Let's just go back to the way it used to be." Godwin shifted her tone from anger and spoke to the board in an apocryphal tone of desperation. "Y'all, we're losing this country, and we're losing it a lot because of how we're handling illegal immigration, and I am just beggin' you—take these things seriously because they are *very* serious." Sitting down next to King, Godwin looked at him and they exchanged smiles and decisive nods. The two of them appeared to think they had been victorious in swaying the board members' minds by using a racist appeal of "losing the country" to immigrants.

Hanley thanked Godwin for her comments. "Kay, thank you for coming—I respect all the work you're doing. . . . Look, you got a friend up here, DA knows he has a friend up here, we're all on the same side, that's why we're here." More than "being on the same side," Hanley suggested he was a similar type of activist to King and Godwin: "I'm not a lawyer; we've got plenty of them up here, and they've done a good job making sure the legal pieces are pretty tangled. Me and the Sheriff are the 'out of control grassroots nutcases,' as they call us in the media, sometimes; so we're on your side, and we've got to selectively make sure we get the ones that are really overstepping the law." Apparently the "out of control grassroots nutcase" was attempting to be more measured and reasonable than Godwin and King.

In a fiery discussion about how to handle King's complaint, DCA representatives asserted again they did not have enforcement powers to demand noncompliant agencies become compliant, and Vinson explained the board could not investigate all 600 entities, suggesting King choose the "worst offenders" and refile his complaints. Godwin and others accompanying King offered services such as printing letters, and one man, Greg Griffin, suggested the board enact a bounty hunter system offering rewards to citizens who identify noncompliant agencies. In other words, Griffin wanted the state of Georgia to put a bounty on the metaphorical heads of its own agencies so citizens could collect on those agencies for not being harsh enough to immigrants. Further, King requested that the board ask the governor for more funding to carry out investigative procedures, and Kent agreed with the idea, asking about its current funding.

"We have the ability to be reimbursed per diem for meetings, get reimbursed for any court reporter, or transcription," Vinson explained, attempting not to detail how much money in particular the board had. Schwinne, sitting in the audience, explained the board had $20,000 annually, prompting Kent to say the board could ask for more money to start traveling and Kent requested a motion for the board to at least double the current budget for enforcement purposes. Schwinne explained that the DoA could not just move money and that the appropriations committee would have to do this.

Requests for growing the IERB budget are deeply ironic. The IERB proposed its publicly financed budget for ensuring undocumented immigrants do not receive public funds be enlarged. Anti-government rhetoric often hinges on economic concerns, as King emphasized when claiming the intent of HB 87 was to "protect jobs." While King and IERB members argued the need to ostensibly protect public funds from being used by immigrants, they simultaneously looked for ways to *extend and increase funded bureaucracy* to ensure undocumented immigrants do not receive any type of publicly financed benefit. For King, Godwin, and Griffin, spending money to make sure immigrants do not receive that money is reasonable and appropriate.

IERB meetings and the relationship among its members, legislators, and immigration opponents like King reveal the challenges in studying governmental power as an anthropologist. These challenges include the difficulty anthropologists can have when trying to study "the state" since the state comprises sets of actors with their own specific agendas who can be influenced by other individuals. The IERB in particular demonstrates challenges in studying the state and governmental power because it is not clear if policy makers and IERB members are taking direction from loud anti-undocumented immigrant protestors like King, if policy makers have their own agendas and pay no attention to people like King, or if there is constant collaboration and communication between government decision makers and anti-immigrant zealots. In public, King claimed to have helped write HB 87 (Swift 2011), and if he had a role in assisting with developing legislation, it is unclear how he obtained this role and was able to continue to serve in it.

The ambiguous ties among King, the IERB, and legislators highlight what sociologist Philip Abrams (1988) has argued: that the state has the ability to prevent adequate study of itself. Similarly, the ability of legislators like Matt Ramsey to avoid researchers is perhaps a product of what anthropologist Hugh Gusterson has called the "cultural invisibility of the rich and powerful" (1997, 115). Legislators are able to shroud their power with forms of secrecy such as ignoring interview requests as Ramsey did. Nevertheless, anthropologists and other social scientists have a duty to study the state, powerful populations, technologies of power like immigration enforcement laws, and their myriad, sometimes hidden, consequences.[5] The secrecy of the state was further emphasized to me when the IERB concluded its March 2013 meeting. As the meeting finished and the board discussed its finances and the need to get more money from the state to conduct investigatory work, another immigration bill, HB 125, which King heavily championed, simultaneously passed in the House.[6]

PASSAGE OF HB 125

HB 125 proposed measures that would prohibit undocumented immigrants from being able to turn on utilities or rent housing. It also excluded foreign passports as acceptable forms of identification to enter government buildings, open bank accounts, enroll children in school, and in some jurisdictions, get married. The Georgia Senate had a similar bill, SB 160, that was proposed and under debate, but excluded elements related to housing. It is not unusual to see similar bills with minor distinguishing differences in each chamber of a legislature, and once the IERB meeting adjourned, I asked Jim what he thought the implications of HB 125 passing were. Since the bill passed in the House, it still had to be adopted in the Senate before making its way to the governor's desk.

"All we can hope now is that the Senate doesn't adopt it. They've got their own version of the bill, SB 160, and we can hopefully change some minds about it and get it at least so people can turn on utilities and rent apartments." Jim spoke with legislators, business representatives, and organization leaders to push for changing SB 160 and HB 125 so they would not bar undocumented immigrants from being able to obtain utilities. "I just can't believe they're still doing this stuff—did they not see the results of the [2012 presidential] election?! It's going to come back to bite them later." As Jim noted, the 2012 presidential election resulted in public discussions about Latinx voters being an important portion of the electorate and immigration concerns being important issues to Latinx voters (Pew Hispanic Center 2012). However, pundits and political officials are wrong to generalize *all* Latinx voters and assume they all vote based on immigration-related issues. As the 2016 election showed, a large number of Latinxs voted for Donald Trump on the basis of perceived shared religious values or owing to a general discontent with existing politics (Khalid 2016).

While SB 160 was being debated, GIRRC organized a group of people to attend a legislative review hearing to comment on the need to amend the bill. On the day of the hearing, I went to the capitol, but when I arrived at the basement room where the hearing was supposed to be held, no one was present. I went upstairs to find Jim frantically walking around talking on his cell phone. I asked Mateo, a GIRRC member there for the hearing, what was going on. "They're about to adjourn until next week," he said. "That'll be a nice break—today is Wednesday and they will start again next Wednesday." As Mateo and I walked down to the elevator bank to make our way back to the hearing room, we met an ACLU attorney also planning on attending the SB 160 hearing. When we entered the hearing room, we noticed handouts for legislation unrelated to SB 160 and two young staffers waited in the room—one sitting, the other standing with a stack of papers.

"Is this the room for the SB 160 hearing?" Mateo asked. A sleepy-eyed staffer from Ramsey's office answered (barely) affirmatively. Another staffer, who had just entered the room and began placing handouts on tables, informed us the hearing had been canceled. "Oh, sweet!" Ramsey's staffer exclaimed, hastily leaving the room. Mateo and I looked at the other staffer incredulously. "Yeah the meeting was canceled but I didn't see anything about it being rescheduled on the agenda," the other staffer added. Mateo asked if there was any additional information about when the hearing would be rescheduled. The staffer did not know, and Mateo thanked him as we left the room. "Fuck! Fuck, fuck, fuck, fuck, fuck!" Mateo exclaimed. "We've got to call everybody and tell them that this thing is canceled." Mateo and I went upstairs to the ground floor of the capitol and walked outside to begin calling GIRRC members to notify them the hearing had been canceled. I met up with Jim later in the day to find out why the SB 160 meeting was canceled, and we rode down the elevator together to the back exit of the building.

When Jim and I found a place to sit, I asked him about the SB 160 meeting. "I knew the meeting would be canceled so that they could reschedule it and hope that not as many people could attend. They knew that we raised awareness about the bill so now they're going to reschedule and find time when not as many people can make it." That was the Republican counterstrategy to activism against their bill: cancel the meeting that everyone knew about and reschedule the meeting so people would have a hard time coming back to the capitol. The idea of an open government accessible to constituents was clearly not alive and well in Georgia. When constituents demanded to be heard, government representatives strategized to ignore their voices and move forward with their agenda. The canceled meeting further pointed to another way in which the state can conceal itself and prevent it from being studied effectively.

After Jim and I talked about the SB 160 fiasco, we discussed which legislators I could interview since Ramsey and other Republicans kept avoiding me. He again told me it was unlikely that Republicans, including Ramsey and other co-sponsors of Georgia's immigration laws, would speak to me. "If you were from Fox News," Jim laughed, "then maybe you'd have a shot!" Ultimately I never interviewed

Ramsey or any Georgia Republicans—all of them denied my meeting requests. The Georgia legislature eventually passed SB 160, and by the time it was signed into law, it was altered to remove utility restrictions. Nevertheless, SB 160 banned passports as secure forms of identification in certain circumstances, such as applying for public benefits.

UNDERSTANDING IMMIGRANT POLICING: RACE AND CITIZEN PROJECTS

The IERB meetings, interviews with legislators, and participant observation experiences at the capitol point to policy makers' rationalizing immigration legislation like HB 87 through themes of economy, race, and governmental authority. In interviews with legislators, economic scapegoating surfaced as a major explanation for why laws like HB 87 passed. Abrams and other legislators suggested economic scapegoating of immigrants was part of the rationale for passing HB 87 and other immigration laws. Further, in speaking to the IERB, King similarly explained economic reasons behind Georgia's immigration laws. However, economic explanations fail to capture the entirety of the rationale for laws like HB 87 and specifically ignore racial notions of otherness that informed law.

Political efforts to restrict Latinx settlement in suburban Atlanta and access to social services demonstrate anxiety over losing the "whiteness" of the area. Although Atlanta was a prominent hub of the U.S. civil rights movement, it has a history of racial discrimination and segregation. For example, when Georgia's black middle class grew in the early twentieth century, elected officials expanded Jim Crow policies in an effort to assert white dominance (Mixon 1997). In 1906, gubernatorial candidates campaigned on disenfranchising black voters, and tense racial relationships turned violent when white rioters vandalized black-owned businesses and invaded black neighborhoods with guns. At the end of a two-day race riot in 1906, more than one hundred people were killed or wounded (Mixon 1997). Moreover, following desegregation of neighborhoods and public spaces in Atlanta, the city saw a pattern of white flight like that of other major metropolitan areas as white residents left Atlanta for the surrounding suburbs (Odem 2008, 116). Accordingly, the changes to suburban neighborhoods associated with an influx of immigrants I described in the previous chapter are set in a context of long-standing racial inequality.

These conditions are not exclusive to Georgia, however, nor is anti-immigrant rhetoric that focuses on race or "losing the country," as Godwin described. As Chavez (2008) argues, the "Latino threat narrative" is pervasive across the United States and hinges on notions of protecting whiteness. Laws like HB 87, and immigrant policing initiatives generally, demonstrate efforts to uphold racial inequalities through legislation and police action (Roberts 2007). Just as Dorothy Roberts

(2007, 263) writes of the criminal justice system and its way to perpetuate racial inequalities among African Americans, police terror and legislation targeting immigrants are ways to support white supremacy.

The racial and economic logics for legislators passing immigration laws like HB 87 suggest a biopolitical "race war logic," following Foucault's (2003) understanding of race as a way to divide populations. Policies that blame immigrants for high unemployment and punish them for criminality can allow for their "political death" and economic failure in order to support the success of white populations. After all, as Godwin believes, she and other white folks in Georgia are "losing the country" to immigration, and Hanley is "sickened" by immigration when he's on roadways. So under their logic, something must be done to presumably ensure *their* success and not immigrants'.

Although laws like HB 87 may not be fully enforced in some contexts, as Abrams described using the agricultural industry as an example, they nevertheless promote fear among undocumented immigrants, as I describe in more detail in the following chapter. The unenforceability of some immigrant policing measures suggests how policies may be used to symbolically express social discontent, particularly a "dual hostility," as immigration scholar Kitty Calavita calls it, "towards immigrants and government" (1996, 297). Immigrant policing efforts are thus ways of channeling acceptable forms of nativism that purport to address economic and federal government failures.

While lawmakers who supported efforts like HB 87 were offered an opportunity to provide their own accounts of why they thought such legislation was necessary, they all declined. As I have described, the challenges in reaching Republican lawmakers speak to the difficulties associated with ethnography that traces political power. Although studying power and the state may be difficult, it is nevertheless possible to study agents of the state, like lawmakers. Some lawmakers' rationale behind laws like HB 87 reveals how immigrant policing can be understood as what Rose and Novas call "citizenship projects," or ways in which "authorities [think] about (some) individuals as potential citizens [or noncitizens], and the ways they [try] to act upon them" (2008, 439). In Georgia, legislators used HB 87 to engage a race-war discourse and improve political perceptions of the legislators who were seen as "tough on immigration." As some legislators suggested, harsh immigration laws were politically helpful to the legislators who supported them, demonstrating how politicians can construct undocumented immigrants not just as racialized others, but as politically convenient targets of policy. Further, legislation that targets certain populations can also take on new life and morph into new realities, as best demonstrated by the IERB extending funding to the board to carry out its mission.

Regardless of legislators' rationales for immigrant policing measures like HB 87 and SB 160, such policies have negatively impacted some undocumented immigrants, especially when combined in places like metropolitan Atlanta, where

Secure Communities exists alongside 287(g) programs and HB 87. In Georgia, the combination of state statutes and federal immigration policies has altered immigrants' mobility (Stuesse and Coleman 2014; Kline 2018a), as I described in this chapter and the introduction, and led to some immigrants feeling intense anxieties and a strong sense of fear. In the next chapter, I show how these anxieties and fears directly shape immigrants' health and where they seek health services.

3 · "WE LIVE HERE IN FEAR"

Policing, Trauma, and a Shadow Medical System

> Georgia has gone out of its way to be as unfriendly to the undocumented as possible.
>
> —Georgia House Minority Leader Stacey Abrams

One evening I drove to meet Martina at her apartment in Doraville, an Atlanta suburb. Doraville is located along Buford Highway, one of the main thoroughfares along which many immigrants live, and the Latinx population accounts for approximately fifty-five percent of all Doraville residents (United States Census Bureau, 2019). Doraville has a reputation for aggressive policing. A local newspaper investigation determined the city devotes nearly half of its annual budget to police operations and that Doraville police collect more ticket fines per capita than any other municipality in the Atlanta area (Simmons 2014). One of Martina's friends, Yolanda, was a GLAHRiador, and she suggested I speak to Martina because police routinely set up *retenes* (singular *retén*), or checkpoints, outside her apartment. At retenes, officers stop drivers and ask to see their license, making checkpoints a possible moment of police apprehension for undocumented immigrants. The apartment complex where Martina lived was likely built in the 1970s and comprised numerous dark brick buildings that were mostly occupied but showed signs of neglect, such as chipped paint and broken windows, from whoever owned the complex. When I found Martina's unit, I met her and her friend, who began telling me about difficulties they had with police and how policing impacted their ability to seek health services.

Martina, who is in her late thirties or early forties, came to Georgia in 2005. Before then, she worked as a migrant farmworker, and she moved along the east coast migrant farmworker trail from Florida to Georgia and eventually up to Michigan, picking tomatoes, onions, and cherries. "We may have met before!" I joked, explaining that I had met migrant farmworkers in the Tampa Bay area as part of other research projects focused on farmworker health (Kline 2012, 2010; Carrion et al. 2011; Castañeda et al. 2010), and that I grew up in Michigan. "*Posiblemente* [possibly]," she responded, smiling. Although Martina had migrated for work when she was younger, she decided to stay in Florida during her first pregnancy rather than continue along the migration route she had become familiar with, and eventually a friend suggested she move to Georgia. "After I gave birth to my daughter, my friend said, 'you know, Georgia's climate is nice, and there is work there in the shade,'" she explained. "Because I've been used to planting onions, cutting cherries and apples in Michigan, and doing other things in the field, I was ready for a better job, and my friend told me there were better jobs in Georgia."

Despite coming to Georgia for work and hoping life would be easier, Martina explained her life was eventually complicated by the retenes police organized near her home. Officers routinely set up retenes at the closest intersection of her apartment complex. Echoing the stories Adelina and I heard in rural parts of the state, this type of heightened police activity complicated life for Martina. "They put up retenes here all the time and it's hard to leave. I have to drive to get to work and up here at the corner, they put up checkpoints. . . . I can hear the checkpoints from here." Like other undocumented immigrants, Martina is prohibited from getting a driver's license, and, as I described in previous chapters, being stopped by police while driving without a license could lead to her arrest and eventual deportation.

Checkpoints like the ones that occur outside Martina's apartment operate as road closures that permit police officers to stop every vehicle and ask drivers to show their license. Although these types of checkpoints could theoretically occur anywhere, GLAHRiadores and interviewees noted how they frequently occurred outside predominantly Latinx neighborhoods, shopping complexes, churches, and apartment complexes like Martina's. To avoid the checkpoints, Martina and her neighbors altered their driving behaviors. "We know it's better to not go through there or to just keep going the other way at night or in the afternoon."

In describing checkpoints near her, Martina noted that she feels fortunate to have never been stopped by police, and although she tries to avoid checkpoints, she must still drive out of necessity. "I drive, but it's necessary to drive to work— to get yourself one place to another you have to drive. Up to now, thank god, police have never stopped me. But it's scary because before if you got stopped you could pay a fine and someone would bail you out, but now it's not like that. Now you get stopped and you get deported." I asked Martina why she thought police put up roadblocks at the intersection outside the apartment complex, and she explained police did it because of the Latinx immigrants living in the area. "Because I think they know that there are many Latinos that live there or a lot of Latinos go by there," she explained.

Setting up checkpoints outside Latinx neighborhoods and apartment complexes where Latinx immigrants lived amounted to a racial profiling tactic that ultimately produced a deep sense of fear for Martina and other immigrants I interviewed. As a result of fearing police, Martina has decreased how much she drives, especially since she felt the frequency of checkpoints had increased from when she first moved to Georgia. "You drive in fear because you know the police can stop you. . . . So now you only leave the house for what's necessary, not like before when you could go shopping, or go out just to spend time out. If you go out, it's because you have to buy food or go to the store, or get a necessity. It's not like it was before when you could go out whenever you wanted to."

The intensity of immigrant policing tactics ultimately resulted in immigrants like Martina avoiding grocery stores and running errands altogether from behind the wheel of a car. As anthropologist Catherine Lutz (2014) has argued, cars are a central feature of mobility in the United States, and a lack of car-based mobility can heighten social inequalities. In Atlanta, immigrant policing directly impacts some immigrants' willingness to get behind the wheel of a car, constraining their mobility (Stuesse and Coleman 2014; Kline 2018a). Moreover, Atlanta lacks a robust public transportation network, making automobiles a necessity for navigating the city, underscoring how racially profiling drivers, specifically, is a strategic way of deploying police as part of an aggressive immigration enforcement regime.

Because some immigrants avoided driving, some local businesses that felt the negative economic impacts of immigrant policing began offering a shuttle service for immigrant customers (see figure 5). As one Doraville grocery store owner explained, "When there are checkpoints, we lose a lot of business. People don't want to come into the store." Moreover, some immigrants began using tools like PaseLaVoz (Pass It On), a text message service that notifies subscribers of nearby reported checkpoints. A driver who sees a checkpoint or police activity can text PaseLaVoz the location and a description of what they saw, and all PaseLaVoz users receive the checkpoint information (Stuesse and Coleman 2014).

Immigrant policing also directly impacted immigrants' health. Martina, like other immigrants I interviewed, explained that she would avoid seeking health services if she thought checkpoints were present, sometimes for long periods of time.[1] For example, over several months, Martina had persistent abdominal pain and nausea, and she would vomit throughout the day. "I was vomiting all the time. . . . My stomach always hurt." She recognized she needed to see a doctor, but she feared that driving to the doctor could expose her to police, resulting in her arrest and possible deportation. When her illness worsened, she decided to risk encountering police to get to a private clinic, and after repeated visits, Martina was eventually diagnosed with hypothyroidism that required specialist care. Although Martina eventually found a way to see a specialist by obtaining a discount card through Grady Memorial Hospital, a public hospital that subsidizes care for residents in two Atlanta counties, Martina worried about leaving her apartment to make her appointments because of the retenes and the authority police had to serve as de facto immigration agents made possible through HB 87. "All these laws are really hard right now, and there have been a lot of laws," Martina

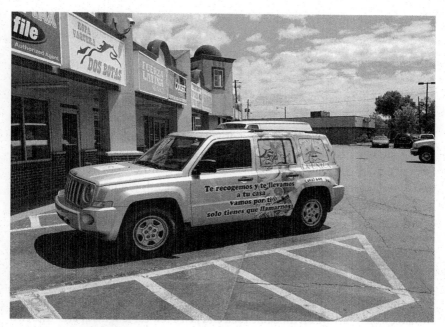

FIGURE 5. A market with a vehicle to transport customers so they do not have to drive. The writing on the vehicle reads "We pick you up and take you back to your house. We'll go for you, all you have to do is call us." (Photo by Nolan Kline.)

explained. "And the police and the checkpoints! It's too much. . . . In other states it's calmer. Here, we live in fear when we leave the house."

Fear of encountering a harsh immigration enforcement regime and intense experiences of racism and exploitation linked to undocumented status have led some immigrants to leave states such as Georgia (Serrano 2012; Associated Press 2010), ultimately harming some states' economies, as I described in the previous chapter. For some undocumented immigrants, immigration laws and police practices have instilled feelings of fear, led to changing mobility and driving practices, and intensified feelings of racial discrimination. But the fear Martina and others experience is not an accidental byproduct of immigration enforcement laws. Instead, fear resulting from immigrant policing is an intentional form of controlling immigrants that not only affects their mobility (see Kline 2018a) but also results in trauma and anxiety. In this chapter, I show how fear is used as a biopolitical technique to attempt to control Latinx immigrants, and I describe how immigration enforcement regimes produce trauma and alter some immigrants' health behaviors. Moreover, I discuss how immigrant policing ultimately created a demand for what I call a "shadow medical system": a patchwork of clandestine health services fraught with potential for exploitability and medical harm.[2] To demonstrate why a shadow medical system emerged in Atlanta and why policing affected some immigrants' health behaviors, I first start with describing how immigrant policing created a heightened sense of fear and trauma among some immigrants, which in some cases had somatic manifestations.

STRESS, TRAUMA, AND IMMIGRANT POLICING

As Martina indicated, police intimidation had several consequences for some immigrants, which included avoiding driving. Moreover, specific police practices like checkpoints resulted in significant stress for some immigrants. For example, Palomita and her family moved from the Atlanta exurb of Forest Park to a town thirty minutes south of Atlanta because police frequently put up retenes near their home and outside their church.[3] "You would leave [the service] and they would be there outside the parking lot, waiting," a friend of Palomita's who still lived in Forest Park recalled. Shortly after they moved, Palomita and her family noticed police organizing retenes outside their new home. "They started putting up retenes right here along this road," Palomita said, gesturing to the two-lane road outside her home. "It was worse than where we used to live because there's only one exit from the neighborhood." Palomita lives in a trailer park where there are two entrances, but both are off the same road and just a few car lengths apart. "The two exits would be blocked—one [police car] on the left and one on the right. . . . They did this daily. Not a single day of rest." The frequency of the retenes created significant stress for Palomita. "It really traumatized us because we could not even leave."

The kind of trauma related to intense policing that Palomita described points to how state-created terror works. In his ethnographic accounts of fear and violence in Northern Ireland, Allen Feldman (1991) indicates how the body itself becomes a terrain where politics play out and the fear of encountering agents of the state results in new articulations of control. For immigrants in Atlanta, terror has several types of results: some immigrants, such as Esme, became hypervigilant while driving and frequently inspected their vehicles, and others felt the embodied consequences of immigrant policing, as I describe below. Hypervigilance, like driving with extraordinary caution, inspecting vehicles, avoiding police, and not leaving the house, points to how some immigrants internalized immigrant policing efforts.

Adding to the stress of being stopped by police was the financial stress associated with being apprehended at a checkpoint, and Palomita described how checkpoints proved profitable for law enforcement agencies. Some days, officers would arrest multiple people at checkpoints for driving without a license. "They saw there was money to be made," Palomita asserted. "The ticket for driving without a license was $1,000 for each person; there were times they got 10–14 people. . . . Imagine you stop 10 people at a reten in one hour—that's $10,000." The retenes were more than a money-making scheme, however, and were part of an overall racist set of policies and police actions. "This is racism. Discrimination against Latinos," Palomita affirmed.

One day, Palomita found GLAHR's information; fed up with the retenes, she wanted to take action, so she called Adelina to ask for help. Palomita, Adelina, and one of Palomita's neighbors scheduled a meeting where more than one hundred people in the neighborhood came to discuss the retenes. At the meeting, they organized a march to the local police station, where Adelina and Don Teo met with station leaders and demanded they stop the checkpoints outside the trailer park. "The police lied," Palomita explained. "They said they did one reten a month—they did 28 a month." Although police continued putting up checkpoints after the meeting, Palomita noticed a decrease in their frequency. To reduce the effect of the remaining retenes, Palomita and her friend began putting up flags near the trailer park exit when they saw police as a way to notify people before they left the neighborhood, and they started a text message chain notifying people of police presence. These strategies, Palomita believed, ultimately led police to abandon the retenes, and when we met, there had not been a checkpoint outside her neighborhood in six months.

Palomita's experience underscores the type of intimidation that occurs with immigrant policing and how the presence of enforcement increased immigrants' fears, led to financial exploitation, and limited their movement. As she described, this type of intimidation traumatized her and her family members because police were constantly outside their home and they felt they could not leave. Eventually, Palomita, her neighbors, and Adelina fought against the intense checkpoint system in their community, but this type of aggressive policing and its resultant trauma was not unusual for many immigrants in Atlanta. Moreover, the intensity of policing and checkpoints amplified fears and trauma among some immigrants.

Ariana, a young undocumented woman from Mexico, sat on a couch in her home across from me. "You can't know what it's like," she said with tears rolling down her face. "The worst part of all these immigration laws is being afraid all the time—I get into my car and I start shaking. If I see a police car, I start crying because I know they could stop me, I could get arrested and deported, and never see my kids again." Ariana was born in Mexico but came to the United States with her parents when she was a child. She described how immigration laws directly affected her by producing a deep sense of fear. "The worst part of all of this is the constant feeling of fear; I'm afraid to leave my house. I'm afraid of the police so I just don't go out. The fear never stops, and it's so bad that I shake when I drive." Ariana continued: "I feel traumatized. All these laws make me feel like I have post-traumatic stress or something. That's what it feels like—trauma. Every day I leave the house but I'm not sure I'll return. It's horrible to live with this constant fear."

Ariana's experience of feeling post-traumatic stress and the anxieties associated with immigrant policing underscore what several anthropologists and epidemiologists have argued in other contexts: that the social world in which we live can impact our bodies and metaphorically "get under our skin" (McEwen 2012; Hertzman and Boyce 2010; Gravlee 2009; Lende and Lachiondo 2009). In Ariana's case, immigrant policing as a social phenomenon can lead to a stress response like anxiety or, as she put it, post-traumatic stress. In recent years, the traumatogenic consequences of immigration enforcement regimes have been increasingly well documented. Public health scholars, for example, have shown how home raids can result in symptoms that fit the diagnostic criteria for post-traumatic stress disorder, including suicidality and inability to care for children (Lopez, Novak et al. 2018). Like raids, immigrant policing efforts produce trauma among those they target, but differ from raids in that they are chronic social conditions that erode immigrants' health over time.

Shaking while driving and crying at the sight of a patrol car demonstrate the somatic consequences of policies designed to instill fear. Migration scholar Sarah Willen observed similar situations among undocumented immigrants in Israel fearing deportation. Willen (2007b, 16) notes that fear resulted in a "persistent, embodied tension and anxiety" and insecurity among some undocumented immigrants, evident in their bodily motions. These motions included moving their heads in multiple directions to look for police while navigating public spaces as part of an effort to stay attentive to police presence. Such actions demonstrate how, as Feldman argues, political terror can be "sunk into the lived body" (1997b, 50), and in the case of some immigrants, expressed through anxiety. In Atlanta, immigrant policing creates a form of terror that some immigrants feel the moment they enter a car, and they not only search for police while driving but immediately think of the consequences of what police presence may bring, like being separated from children, as Ariana noted.

The physiological responses some immigrants have to the possibility of a police stop demonstrate how immigrant policing is a constant reminder of immigrants' liminal position in the United States and the types of insecurity associated with undocumentedness. For example, one woman, Henriqua, explained that the threat of encountering police and associated risk of deportation not only made her fearful but also made her feel unsafe. "I feel like I live in a warzone," she said. "It's never safe and you have to always be on the lookout. In Mexico, you run the risk of getting kidnapped or killed; here, you run the risk of getting stopped and deported. I'm not safe here, and I'm not safe there—there's nowhere safe for me." For Henriqua, not feeling safe was directly related to the risk of apprehension at any given moment, and immigrant policing efforts construct and operate on this risk.

Feeling unsafe with police further reveals how immigration enforcement erodes immigrants' relationships with law enforcement agents. For example, as immigrant policing efforts intensified in Atlanta, employees at a mental health counseling clinic, the Center for Education, Treatment, and Prevention of Addiction (CETPA), noticed their patients having increasingly negative feelings about police. "There's a lot of hatred," one CETPA provider explained. "They don't see the police anymore as somebody who is going to protect them, but somebody who is going to harm them or punish them." It is no surprise, then, that the Cobb United for Change Coalition (CUCC) members reported that undocumented Latinx immigrants in their neighborhoods hesitated to call law enforcement when they were victims of violent crimes or robberies; and in some locations, thieves made a point of targeting undocumented immigrants as they exited convenience stores after cashing paychecks precisely because immigrants would hesitate to call police owing to their fear of being deported. This kind of predatory theft, combined with distrust of police, undoubtedly contributed to feeling as if "there's nowhere safe" for some undocumented immigrants, like Ariana and Henriqua.

Feeling as if nowhere is safe and having a constant reminder of the potential for deportation are intentional outcomes of immigrant policing efforts. The internalized crises of security that immigrants like Ariana face are part of the design of immigration enforcement regimes comprising laws like HB 87, which attempt to advance an "attrition through enforcement" strategy promoted by some politicians (Kobach 2008). Attrition through enforcement efforts include restricting access to public education, employment, and a variety of social services for undocumented immigrants with the intention of making some immigrants' lives so difficult that they "self-deport" (García 2013). The attrition through enforcement strategy represents a specific form of terrorizing immigrants through political apparatuses and a strategic use of fear to control some immigrants. Given this context, the types of physiological responses immigrants describe, like shaking while driving and crying when seeing police, are a manifestation of trauma that is entirely politically created and intentional.

The psychological and physiological responses some immigrants have to aggressive immigrant policing regimes underscore how fear itself can become a "chronic condition," as anthropologist Linda Green (1994) has described. Policing in Atlanta points to a type of fear and insecurity that persists in individuals' lives and becomes routine. Green discusses overt violence in the wake of governmental unrest—a situation undeniably different from what occurs in immigrant policing contexts like Atlanta. The situation in Atlanta is a subtler way of producing a fear response, masked through the seemingly neutral and innocuous but formal arena of policy and law. Fear-based governance resulting from immigrant policing, then, is a concealed type of terror that nevertheless results in embodied consequences and persistent anxieties. Moreover, the trauma produced from attempts to govern immigrants through fear can translate to poor mental health outcomes and increased potential for substance abuse among some immigrants.

IMMIGRANT POLICING, DEPRESSION, AND ANXIETY

In their examination of chronic conditions, anthropologists Lenore Manderson and Carolyn Smith-Morris (2010, 18) demonstrate how long-term health conditions are increasingly linked to political and economic circumstances. They specifically draw attention to how political factors are implicated in continual health concerns. Similarly, in Atlanta, immigrants and providers alike have identified immigrant policing as a political etiology of some mental health concerns and in some instances, substance abuse.

Pointing to the persistent consequences of immigration enforcement regimes, one mental health provider explained how some of her immigrant patients have developed long-term depression. "They're just so depressed and feel hopeless," she explained. "They feel like they can't do the normal things in life they'd like to do." Adding to this, she noted that feeling hopeless is a risk factor for alcohol abuse. "We know that people will self-medicate [using alcohol as an escape], and right now we're seeing people use alcohol because of all these immigration laws." For example, one man, Esteban, explained that his friends and neighbors who were also undocumented started to drink more than they did in the past. "Ever since all these laws and things, I see them going out, getting drunk, and coming back home late. The drinking has gotten really bad, and it's because of all these laws." Esteban further explained immigrant policing and alcohol use through a gendered analysis, asserting that immigrant policing limited his and other men's ability to drive for work, restricting their economic contributions to their households and resulting in frustration that led some men to abuse alcohol. "When men can't work and can't provide for their families, it upsets us, and I see a lot of people deal with that by drinking." As I describe in the next chapter, immigrant policing led some men to abuse alcohol as a coping mechanism, but the alcoholism resulted in other deleterious health consequences, such as intimate partner violence. Esteban's comments about alcohol abuse point to how immigrant policing can create gendered health-related experiences and reinforce gendered expectations of economically providing for family members. His assertion about men as providers, however, merits critique. During my time in Atlanta, many of the women I met were sole providers for their households, including Anita, to whom I return in the next chapter.

At CETPA, providers and staff echoed Esteban's association of substance abuse with immigrant policing and fears of encountering police. CETPA provides substance abuse prevention and treatment services and mental health counseling for Latinx populations. The organization opened in 1999 and has three overall branches of service: prevention, intervention, and treatment. Prevention services target Latinx youth aged ten to seventeen and include bilingual curriculums delivered at various organizations and institutions around Georgia focused on alcohol and drug use, depression, self-esteem, nutrition, suicidal ideation, pregnancy, and bullying. Intervention services include a clubhouse where Latinx youth meet after school to focus on homework and participate in programs focused on similar topics covered by the prevention services. The clubhouse also provides space for youth who are at risk of getting kicked out of school to receive tutoring and other services to improve their educational outcomes. CETPA's treatment services are the largest component of the organization, serving over 400 children and adults through nearly 20 clinical staff.

One CETPA staff member, who had worked at the organization since the early 2000s, explained that several new patients started coming to CETPA for treatment of anxiety, depression, and substance abuse related to immigration enforcement. "We have a lot of clients coming to our clinic because they started getting really anxious and depressed because of these laws and all the checkpoints." These clients sought treatment because of how immigrant policing amplified anxieties about housing, economic, and familial instability. "We have a lot of clients saying, 'I don't know what to do; do I have to leave the country? . . . My husband has to go out every day and he has to drive but he doesn't have a driver's license and I don't know what's going to happen right now. If he has to stop working, and I have two or three kids, how are we going to feed them?'" This staff member frequently heard this type of scenario but noted that some patients ceased services. "These were the ones coming in, though. A lot of patients [we had been seeing already] stopped coming because of these laws and because they were too afraid to drive."

As the CETPA staff member's comment suggests, and as Martina suggested earlier, fear of encountering police could also result in immigrants avoiding social and health services (see Alexander and Fernandez 2014). As Ariana explained, "It's just not safe to drive, not even if I'm sick. What would I do if they stopped me? Who would take care of my children?" Avoiding health services in situations of medical need underscores how immigrant policing regimes employ fear as a mechanism of control, or as Foucault (1977) calls it, "a technology" of governing immigrants. The CETPA staff member argued that in some situations, some patients may even cease certain types of treatment they already started. Immigrant policing efforts interfere with whether someone might seek treatment for a specific, acute health issue, and also whether the individual could continue treatment for continuous health concerns. Nevertheless, some situations necessitated medical intervention, leading some immigrants to find treatment while also avoiding Atlanta's aggressive immigrant policing regime.

FINDING ALTERNATE AVENUES OF CARE

Along Buford Highway, drivers pass numerous immigrant-owned restaurants and businesses in strip malls and shopping complexes such as Plaza Fiesta, where several of GLAHR's popular education events took place. These businesses provide evidence of Atlanta's increasingly diverse immigrant population (Odem 2008, 115). In addition to serving as a location for restaurants and shops, Buford Highway, smaller connecting roads, and other areas with high concentrations of immigrant residents also serve as locations for small Latinx clinics that some immigrants considered safe from police. These clinics typically had signs in Spanish with names such as Clínica Latina[4] and advertised to Latinx patients in local Spanish-language periodicals. For many immigrants, these clinics were considered safe because they would not ask for forms of documentation that would reveal a patient's immigration status, like a social security number or driver's license.

Asking for certain types of identification can spark significant stress for someone like Martina, who lives with the constant threat of deportation. Not having needed information can also result in being denied certain services. For example, when Martina went to Grady Memorial Hospital for her hypothyroidism, she had to apply for a Grady Card, the discount card that would allow her to receive subsidized care. To receive a Grady Card, an applicant must provide a government-issued ID, such as a passport, social security card, or driver's license; proof of residence; proof of income; and proof of family size. Despite bringing required documentation, however, Martina was initially unable to get the card. "When I tried to get the card, the [staff member] asked me for a Social Security number and driver's license, and I told her that I didn't have a license or a Social Security number." Because Martina did not have the requested documentation, the staff member denied her a Grady Card. "She wouldn't give me the card because I didn't have a license or social security number! I can't get a license!" Frustrated with her situation, Martina asked for an interpreter at the hospital and told him she did not have a license but had a Mexican passport. "[The interpreter] gave me a [Grady] card with the passport," she explained. Martina fought for a medical discount card, and the same situation that makes her vulnerable to arrest—being undocumented and not being allowed to have a driver's license—made her susceptible to a capricious decision from a hospital staff member to not accept her passport as valid identification.

Reflecting on why the interpreter gave her a Grady Card but the first staff member would not, Martina felt as if she had been discriminated against because she is Latinx. "It's racism or something, or maybe because I don't speak the language, but the lady [at Grady] didn't want to give me the card. I showed her my passport and she told me that she wanted a Georgia driver's license and I told her I don't have a license. I think it's racism." As Martina's experience shows, being undocumented in a clinical setting can result in arbitrary application of rules, like demanding a Georgia driver's license to secure a medical discount card. These moments can, as Martina suggested, serve as reminders of racism and inequality. Additionally, being asked for a license or social security number can serve as a reminder of the insecurity associated with undocumentedness. This type of insecurity, and the type of terror associated with police tactics, can contribute to persuading immigrants to seek services from the small Latinx clinics along and near Buford Highway or in other immigrant neighborhoods. Avoiding police and institutional scrutiny is why one undocumented woman, Sandra, chose to go to Latinx clinics.

Sandra was in her early twenties when we met, and she came to Atlanta when she was twelve. Sandra's mother moved to Atlanta when Sandra was nine to help support the family. "It was really, really hard," Sandra said. "We don't have a dad, and [my mom] was working, but it was not enough money to feed four kids and my grandma." Once Sandra finished her elementary education, her mother sent a friend to Mexico to bring Sandra to Georgia. The first time she tried to cross, Sandra walked for three days and three nights with a group. "There were like 50 people, and I was the youngest there, and it was all males. We had to sleep on a mountain." On the fourth day, border patrol apprehended Sandra, fingerprinted her, and deported her to Mexico. "I was so scared and crying," Sandra recalled. But, as she told me, "a few days later, we tried again." The second time she tried to cross, Sandra and her mother's friend were successful, and they made it to Tucson, Arizona, without encountering immigration officials and survived the arduous journey that often results in migrants' deaths (De León 2015).

Sandra finished high school in Georgia and wanted to go to college. She had the grades to get into any of Georgia's universities, but because she is undocumented, she is ineligible to attend state-funded universities and cannot get student loans to help finance her education, making her college goals difficult to achieve. When we talked about where she goes for health services, Sandra explained that she prefers to visit a Latinx clinic when sick. "I go to Clínica de las Americas if I'm sick." Sandra noted that at the clinic she may not receive the correct treatment and may overpay for the services she receives, but she knows she will not encounter the kinds of misunderstandings Martina described. "You may pay more and they may not give you the right medicine, but I just feel more comfortable there. I know it's safe." For Sandra, the feeling of safety was more important than quality of care or cost of care, mirroring comments from other interviewees about wanting to find care in a safe location. As Sandra's mother explained when we met, "We know that there are places where you can go and they won't ask you for a social security number. . . . They'll attend to you without asking you if you have a social security number or not—they just see you and you pay. Those are the places we know are safe." In other words, Sandra and her mother found a sense of safety in places free from the reminder of vulnerability linked to undocumented status.

Although a need for safe forms of health care encouraged Sandra and her mother to seek services at Latinx clinics, some immigrants found alternate forms of care because they feared encountering checkpoints and police. These care methods included purchasing over-the-counter medications from *farmacias* (pharmacies) and seeking services from traditional healers. As one young woman explained to me, "If we're sick we just go to the farmacia at Centro Hispanico. They get shipments in from Mexico so you go and tell the person there what you have and they give you something." Similarly, another woman I met through GLAHR explained that rather than going to a health provider, her first choice in seeking treatment for a specific health condition was a farmacia. "For us, we know from our countries where we come from what's good and what you can take care of without visiting a doctor. You don't need to go to a doctor for everything, so you go there to Centro Hispanico and you ask about something, and you buy it, and they give you what you need. You don't have to go to a doctor." For some situations, some interviewees, such as Sandra, would go to a traditional healer, such as *hueseros* (literally, "bonesetter"), a type of traditional healer. As Sandra explained, "Sometimes I go to Doña Maria, the *huesera*. She gives me this stuff to drink and it tastes nasty but it makes me feel better." Similarly, Julieta, a staff member at CETPA, noted some of the clients at CETPA saw a *curandero*, another type of traditional healer, because they were considered safe spaces for care.

Farmacias and traditional healers such as Doña Maria did not always have every type of desired medical intervention, however. For example, Sandra and her cousin Paula had a hard time finding contraceptive options. During lunch one day at Subway, a popular sandwich chain restaurant, Sandra asked if I knew anything about how to find birth control. "Paula used to take these pills in Mexico, but she stopped when she came here because you need a prescription to get birth control. Well she found this *tienda* [store] where she can get pills that come from Mexico. . . . So I was like 'well that's good, it's easy for us to get the pills.' But I don't like the pill—it causes all these changes in me." Birth control pills can have numerous side effects, and Sandra wanted to prevent pregnancy without the changes she experienced while on medication. "I've heard about the patch, but you have to have a prescription, right? So what can I do?" Neither Sandra nor Paula could find the patch at farmacias, and I suggested she speak with a provider, Dr. Hernandez, whom I met several weeks before our lunch and who specializes in women's health and sexual health. I noted that there were pregnancy prevention methods other than birth control pills or a patch that might work better for Sandra but required a consultation with a physician like Dr. Hernandez. I also referred Sandra and Paula to a website where they could compare contraceptive methods like an intrauterine device and implant, but I was unsure of what else I could do to answer their questions.

Sandra and Paula's difficulties in finding certain types of contraception revealed challenges in relying on farmacias or traditional healers when they were shut out of more formal medical settings because of their undocumented status. Furthermore, their situation revealed how immigrant policing can heighten gendered experiences of what medical anthropologists have described as structural vulnerability: a positionality produced by forms of hierarchization and power differentials based on race, sex, gender, economic status, personal attributes, and other factors (Quesada, Hart, and Bourgois 2011, 340–341). In the United States, women who have sex with men disproportionately carry the burden for pregnancy prevention compared with men who have sex with women (Kimport 2017), and this is true for Sandra and Paula. Added to this gendered expectation, however, is the challenge of finding care from a provider whom the two of them feel is safe, who will see them despite not having insurance, and who will be capable of providing them suitable options to make decisions about their reproductive health that they are comfortable with. In some ways, then, immigrant policing has specific, gendered, health consequences for some women.

In addition to visiting farmacias or traditional healers, some immigrants also visited what I refer to as informal providers, or providers who operate clinics in their garages, on their balconies, or in other parts of their homes. Julieta, an administrator at CETPA, explained that this was a common practice, particularly for seeking oral health services. "Instead of going to a dentist, [some undocumented immigrants] go to somebody with a chair at home," she explained. These providers may have been licensed before moving to the United States, and they continue to practice through informal networks. "Like in Colombia or Mexico, for example, they were dentists and then they come here and they can't do it, so they have to go illegal." Julieta noted that while these providers may not be legally authorized to practice, there is a large cost savings for their patients. "Since it is, for example, $25 for something that would cost $100, people go there. I have done it myself. I had a tooth fixed." Although Julieta's immigration status permitted her access to formal providers, dental care is prohibitively expensive for her, so she decided to seek care from an informal dentist she heard about from her clients. "He had a chair; there was a drill and everything. . . . It is just like being in an office except it is in their dining room or on their porch. Mine was in an enclosed porch in a condo," Julieta added.

Seeking care from Latinx clinics, farmacias, and informal providers was an avenue to care for some immigrants living in Atlanta and needing to avoid aggressive immigrant policing regimes. Some situations, however, required visiting a hospital, but as Sandra explained, "I have to be dying if I'm going to go to the hospital, like *dying*, you know? It's just not worth the risk to go to a doctor if you feel sick." Whereas more than 125 million U.S. residents use hospitals for outpatient services in a year (National Center for Health Statistics 2017), for some immigrants in Georgia, hospitals were last resorts for health care. Relying on alternate sources of care may have been a way for some immigrants to avoid aggressive policing tactics and find care in safe spaces, but some local providers questioned some of these practices and expressed concerns over Latinx clinics, specifically, exploiting patients.

"BLACK MARKET MEDICINE" AND A SHADOW MEDICAL SYSTEM

In discussing the role of Latinx clinics for providing care to some undocumented immigrants, health care providers I spoke with directly expressed concerns over the legitimacy of Latinx clinics and suggested that patients who sought care at them were not treated by "real" or licensed physicians and routinely overpaid for services. Such critiques could be because providers were unhappy with how Latinx clinics and other sources of care potentially threatened the hegemony of biomedical treatment networks, but providers specifically expressed concerns about Latinx clinics having questionable quality, something Sandra noted in describing the clinics she visited. As one provider said, acknowledging that Latinx clinics were comfortable spaces for some immigrants because they would not ask for documentation, "Sure they won't ask you for a social security number, but will they give you the right treatment?" Further, one provider called Latinx clinics "black market medicine."

Although some health providers were suspicious of Latinx clinics, providers' claims about these clinics were difficult to verify without insider knowledge of how all the Latinx clinics operate. There are numerous Latinx clinics around Atlanta, and I am not making sweeping judgments about all of them, but rather I aim to show how some of them may have exploited undocumented patients. For example, news stories shed light on fraudulent activity occurring in some now-defunct Latinx clinics, including one that repeatedly came up in interviews and was highly visible because of its frequent use of billboard advertisements: Clínica de la Mama. The clinic had numerous locations in the Atlanta area, including Plaza Fiesta. I had attempted to interview staff at Clínica de la Mama, but during my efforts, the clinic abruptly and mysteriously shut down. I discovered much later that the clinic was embroiled in a lawsuit for committing Medicaid fraud, and ultimately leaders of the company that operated the clinic admitted to channeling undocumented pregnant patients to specific hospitals for a kickback (McDonald 2014; United States Department of Justice 2014; Weaver 2014).

As part of the clinic's scheme, staff would direct patients to deliver babies at specific hospitals and discourage them from delivering at other locations, suggesting Medicaid may not pay for the deliveries. As I noted in chapter 1, undocumented women are eligible for Emergency Medicaid during their pregnancy. As a result of the clinic funneling patients to certain hospitals, the hospitals participating in the scheme were able to increase their revenue from Georgia's Medicaid program (McDonald 2014). These fraudulent business practices do not necessarily speak to the quality of care provided to patients, but nevertheless suggest that Clínica de la Mama's interests were not entirely aligned with patients', and that some clinic leadership exploited patients for economic gain.

Economic factors were one of the major critiques providers had of Latinx clinics. As one provider at a major hospital, Dr. Samuel, noted, "They're not free clinics but they're clinics where [immigrants] can be seen and feel safe to go to, but they cost them out-of-pocket." To Dr. Samuel, the cost did not justify the lack of quality of care. "I don't know the people staffing those, and I don't know [their] quality . . . but I've seen some badness coming out of there, like sick people who then come to me and I say 'they told you what?!'"

Like Dr. Samuel, Dr. Hernandez, to whom I referred Sandra and Paula, discussed concerns with Latinx clinics. Dr. Hernandez is an OB/GYN with a large Latinx patient population and is a native Spanish speaker who has lived in Atlanta for nearly twenty years. She operates her own OB/GYN practice in association with one of Atlanta's hospitals, and she occasionally participated in a nonprofit Latinx health organization. One of Dr. Hernandez's sources of frustration was how Latinx clinics ended up costing patients more money in the long run because of the poor quality of care they provided. "You have the little clinics that will do the $25 Pap smear, but the problem is that a lot of these clinics do not have specialty doctors, so I see a lot of patients that will come in and bring me stuff that's been given to them and they end up paying *more* because they don't get properly treated," Dr. Hernandez explained. "They keep going [and treatments do not work] and then eventually somebody says 'you need to go to Dr. Hernandez.' So they have wasted all this money on stuff that wasn't going to make them better to begin with." She later added, "A lot of times patients will bring bags of medicines, and they didn't need any of it. And I'll ask, 'well how much did you pay for that one?' [and they will say] 'That was $34 and this one was *cien* [$100].' So there in the bags is the [cost of the] visit where they could've come to me and gotten the right treatment. There're a lot of providers taking advantage [of these patients]."

In some situations, Dr. Hernandez noted that at some clinics, staff may lie to pregnant patients and charge them a cash fee and collect Medicaid fees. "There's one clinic that's really, really famous and the guy that runs it is not even a doctor— Clínica del Sur. If [patients] go there it's because they're afraid to apply for anything [like Medicaid] but they don't understand that the clinic then says 'okay the fee is $500,' but then the office takes it upon themselves to apply for Emergency Medicaid and they'll get the Emergency Medicaid. . . . They make patients sign papers and all that stuff. They do all that and they get terrible care." In this example, the clinic ultimately collects reimbursements for care from Medicaid and collects high fees from patients.

As part of a typical prenatal care regimen, a pregnant woman will visit a provider at least once after delivery. "You are considered to be in a pregnant state until you're six weeks postpartum," Dr. Hernandez explained, noting the importance of a postpartum visit. "That postpartum visit is crucial, and one of the things that I found is that a lot of women came here for just that postpartum visit, saying 'well my doctor said just come here.' And I'm like 'No!'" Dr. Hernandez found it particularly outraging that providers sent patients to her with whom she had no history of working. She said she has to tell them, "We didn't see you for your pregnancy, we don't have any notes about your pregnancy, I don't know whether you had any issues with your pregnancy or not, and for me to just do your postpartum care blindly? No!"

To Dr. Hernandez, poor prenatal care was perhaps the most egregious example of Latinx clinics extorting patients for money. The clinics typically charged a flat fee for a number of visits, but the fee excluded the final postpartum visit. "It used to infuriate me because if you are going to charge them money to take care of their pregnancy that [postpartum] visit should be included even if you have to charge a fee of $100 or $200, but when they call to get their postpartum visit and you just say 'go to the health department'? I think in some ways that there's just some substandard care that they get." In Dr. Hernandez's opinion, this substandard care was due to a lack of patient advocates and limited access to the formal health care treatment network, which was made more difficult to access because of immigrant policing. "Who is guiding them? Who is helping them? Who is deciding what is best for them?" Dr. Hernandez asked me, angered by the situations she sees in her clinic. "And then to be turned away for basic care that should be part of what they do! It's upsetting!"

Dr. Hernandez thought some prenatal care clinics that exploited patients did not have physicians: this included the well-known Buford Highway location of Clínica de la Mama, which she suggested was a place where immigrants did not "get real care." The question of whether patients got "real care" from "real providers" was something that also concerned public health officials. One local health department leader and practitioner who saw a large number of Latinx patients worried about the treatment her patients got. "I've had Hispanic women come in and their blood pressure is through the roof," she explained. "They have a history of high blood pressure and they say, 'well I was on blood pressure medication until last year,' and I will ask 'why did you stop?' [and they will say] 'Well my doctor said I was cured.' And I tell them, 'you are cured because you're on the medication—did you ever go back after you stopped?' 'No, no, he just said I didn't have to take it anymore.'" Situations like this raised numerous concerns for this official, including whether the providers had medical backgrounds.

In questioning the quality of Latinx clinics (see figure 6 for an example of a closed Latinx clinic), Dr. Hernandez also provided examples of seeing patients whom received poor care for concerns other than pregnancy. "Sometimes I see patients that are being treated for early cervical cancer by these clinics and they don't even do LEEP [a common cervical cancer procedure] on them," she said, shaking her head as she spoke.[5] She added that the providers at some Latinx clinics failed to follow proper diagnosis and treatment procedures with cervical cancer patients who ultimately came to her after receiving inappropriate care. "So then

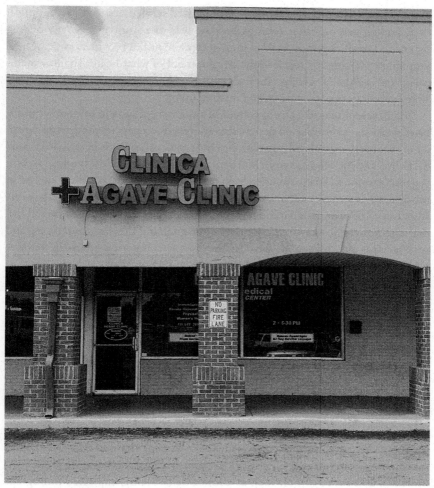

FIGURE 6. An example of a Latinx clinic no longer in operation. (Photo by Nolan Kline.)

I get them in and of course [the other provider] found out that they have [cervical cancer], and they discover it's a little bit more involved and at that point it's like 'oh go here' and they send them to me." This raised questions about providers' training to Dr. Hernandez: "[Just] because a person technically does these procedures does not make them an OB/GYN; they're just people who go to one course, just like if I were to go to one course and then start."

Collectively, immigrants' and providers' experiences demonstrate that there are numerous economic and personal reasons that inform undocumented immigrants' health care decisions, and immigrant policing is one of them. Fears of possible deportation and presence of police who apprehend immigrants inform a risk calculation in which potentially substandard services may be a safer option than finding care in other settings because it is free from aggressive policing regimes. Overall, experiences from immigrants and health providers indicate how immigrant policing has fostered the development of what I call a shadow medical system in Atlanta, which comprises multiple types of care associated with possible exploitation, poor quality, and mistreatment.

The development of a shadow medical system in Atlanta follows other models of multi-tiered health care designed to address discrepancies in types and quality of care for marginalized populations (Mor et al. 2004; Wyss et al. 1996; Frank, McGuire, and Newhouse 1995). In Atlanta, the resulting shadow medical system suggests treatment inequalities exist in part because of fear of using one tier of medical services may result in encountering an aggressive policing regime. In some situations, undocumented immigrants may be eligible for subsidized care at formal care networks, like Grady Memorial Hospital, but they may avoid care and seek services at Latinx clinics because they fear encountering police. In this scenario, a shadow medical system has developed not because of a lack of access but rather because of a need for a health services option that is perceived as safe and less likely to be associated with risks of encountering police. Although fear of the discovery of undocumented status factors into immigrants' health decisions when seeking health services (Heyman, Núñez, and Talavera 2009; Berk 2001; Asch et al. 1998), the Atlanta situation shows how immigrant policing may heighten worries over personal safety and result in some immigrants relying on a potentially poorer quality care network.

While seeking care from Latinx clinics that are considered "safe" for undocumented immigrants can be considered a resistance effort to immigrant policing and a way to resist biomedical hegemony, I hesitate to refer to this type of care as resistance because of insufficient evidence indicating that the quality of care is acceptable. On the contrary, some evidence, including interviewees' experiences, indicates that some clinics, such as Clínica de la Mama, exploited immigrant patients. Rather than being a way to resist immigrant policing, a shadow medical system may directly contribute to immigrants' exploitation and deepen health inequalities.

CHANGING HEALTH BEHAVIORS

As I described earlier in this chapter, immigrant policing efforts like retenes influenced some immigrants' willingness to drive, including in situations of medical need. Moreover, in at least one circumstance, immigrant policing directly altered a preventive health behavior for one immigrant I met, Rosa. One of the GLAH-Riadores introduced me to Rosa, and I scheduled an interview with her over text messages where we confirmed the location and time of the interview. One morning, Rosa sent me a series of text messages asking whether police can stop someone for walking along the street. She repeatedly asked if walking on the street was a crime, and explained that a police car had started following her. When Rosa and I met in person, we talked about the text messages and the patrol car that followed her that morning.

Rosa is in her fifties and has rheumatoid arthritis, which causes joint swelling and pain. If left untreated, inflammation related to the disease can cause joint deformities and bone deterioration. To alleviate some of her arthritis-related pain, Rosa tried to lose weight and regularly exercise. "My doctor recommended I go for walks," she explained, because walking is a low-impact exercise. "I try to go for walks every day." Rosa lives in suburban Cobb County, and her husband provides the main source of income for their family. On the day she sent me text messages about a patrol car following her while she was walking, Rosa feared she would be arrested during her exercise routine. "I didn't know if it was against the law to walk or not—can they arrest me for walking?" Walking is not a crime, but under HB 87, police are empowered to stop Rosa if they suspect she is undocumented. Despite recognizing the need to exercise, Rosa explained that police practices may stop her from engaging in her preventive health routine. "I walk because my doctor recommended it. . . . If the police start following me around all the time, I won't be able to go out anymore. How will I exercise?"

In addition to exercising, Rosa manages her arthritis pain and inflammation by regularly receiving cortisone injections that cost $2,200 a month. Constant pain prevents Rosa from working, but her husband, Eduardo, earns enough to cover the treatment costs. Eduardo explained they could not receive this type of care in the part of Mexico where they are from. "Here she can get the treatment she needs." When we met, Rosa and Eduardo were unsure of how they might continue to get treatment for Rosa's arthritis. Eduardo had been arrested for driving without a license, and his immigration status was discovered. He had recently been issued a deportation notice. "We have to stay here for Rosa's treatment," Eduardo emphasized. "She can't get the injections and it's not safe—if I opened a store or something in Mexico, we'd have to pay $200 a month just to protect us from people who might threaten us."

Rosa and Eduardo's story exemplifies how fear of encountering police can ultimately lead to changing a preventive health behavior. Rosa had engaged in provider-recommended exercise but contemplated ceasing her exercise regimen because of immigrant policing tactics, which in this situation amounted to a patrol car following her in her neighborhood. Her experience reveals how immigrant policing undermines broad public health goals focused on individual health, like routine exercise, and underscores how immigration itself is a social determinant of health (Castañeda, Holmes et al. 2015). While some people might argue that individuals must "be responsible for their health," drawing on neoliberal discourses of individual responsibility, someone like Rosa has a constrained ability to manage her health because immigrant policing efforts made her exercise regimen a risk factor for deportation.

Other types of changes I have discussed in this chapter that some immigrants made because of police also fit into a larger rubric of altering preventive health behaviors. Avoiding seeking care, as Martina or patients at CETPA did, for example, demonstrates how immigrant policing itself is a risk factor for poor health. A CETPA provider emphasized this when noting that some patients stopped seeking services because of checkpoints and roadblocks, or because services occurred at night, when police were more likely to be out. "Clients will tell me 'oh, well I know I need it, but I can't come every week.' Or 'I can't come to the group because the group is at night time and I'm scared to drive in the nighttime because that's when I can get stopped and arrested and I'm really, really scared.'" Similarly, one undocumented interviewee explained, "Driving at night is too risky. We don't leave the house after 10:00 pm because there are too many police around. It doesn't matter if you're sick, if you need medicine—nothing. It's too risky to leave the house."

Some CETPA patients took taxis to their appointments to get needed services but avoid the risk of police detection and deportation. This strategy, however, exacerbated the costs associated with seeking care. As a CETPA provider explained, some patients will walk where they need to go, but not everyone can walk to CETPA. "In one family, one woman walks to church every day and then she walks to three different schools to pick up her kids and then she walks home because she won't drive. But [to come here] they have to pay a taxi or ask a friend." The cost of the taxi or payment to a friend as a thank-you ultimately contributes to the overall cost of their visit, exacerbating cost as a barrier to care. "So it's even more expensive to get medical care. . . . We try to offer low cost services but then they have to pay for a taxi!" As experiences from CETPA providers and immigrants like Rosa show, immigrant policing can directly shape specific individual health behaviors, like engaging in daily exercise or seeking preventive health services.

NEOLIBERAL CITIZENS, THE BIOPOLITICS OF CAUTION, AND BELIED CARE

As immigrants' and health providers' experiences demonstrate, immigrant policing efforts attempt to control immigrants' movement, health care decisions, and feelings of safety by producing fear. Fear, then, is a biopolitical technology of control and a purposeful byproduct of legislation aimed to encourage "immigrant attrition." Such efforts are traumatogenic and ultimately result in a shadow medical system characterized by exploitability and dubious quality. This system can intensify gender and racial inequalities, as exemplified by Sandra's concerns about finding a contraceptive method that best suits her needs, Clínica de la Mama exploiting pregnant women, and Martina's encounter with a Grady staff member arbitrarily choosing to exclude passports as an acceptable form of identification for receiving a hospital discount card. Fear as a mechanism of control does not occur in isolation, but instead operates in tandem with other types of vulnerabilities.

As medical anthropologists have argued, undocumented Latinx immigrants in the United States are subjected to economic exploitation and discrimination based on their sex, gender, and race that occur in conjunction with forms of symbolic violence and assertions that they do not belong in the United States (Quesada, Hart, and Bourgois 2011). These numerous forces that converge and constitute structural vulnerability have resulted in Latinx immigrants occupying a "quasi-caste status in the US" (Quesada, Hart, and Bourgois 2011, 6). Immigrant policing contributes to this quasi-caste system by serving as a reminder of immigrants' deportability and by using law and policy to emphasize immigrants' insecure social status.

In describing undocumented immigrants' numerous vulnerabilities in the United States because of their documentation status, immigration scholar Nicholas De Genova argues that undocumentedness itself is a way to legally construct immigrants' vulnerability to subordinate them (2002, 429). Immigration status becomes a justification for punitive measures and restricting rights. Adding to this idea and focusing on immigration enforcement policies, social scientists Julie Dowling and Jonathan Xavier Inda have argued that U.S. immigration policies specifically "govern immigrants through crime" or "make crime and punishment the institutional context in which efforts to guide the conduct of immigrants take place" (Inda and Dowling 2013, 2). Governing immigrants through crime serves as a way to use law enforcement, the criminal justice system, and even political discourse to cast immigrants as criminal others and work to guide immigrants' conduct.

In Atlanta, immigrant policing regimes not only govern immigrants through crime but also function in ways to guide immigrants' individual health decisions. Immigrant policing efforts ultimately encourage immigrants to be self-sufficient in finding sources of health care rather than relying on state-funded entities. For example, rather than immediately seeking care at state-funded hospitals like Grady, Sandra and other immigrants described how they typically sought care elsewhere, avoiding state-funded institutions to avoid police. This avoidance—a strategy necessitated by harsh immigrant policing regimes—demonstrates how immigrant policing efforts construct a specific kind of citizenship that reinforces neoliberal ideals of self-sufficiency and limited government involvement.

As an economic philosophy, neoliberalism encompasses values such as shrinking state services while simultaneously promoting discourses of individual responsibility to encourage people to provide for themselves rather than seek assistance from the state (Harvey 2007; Hyatt 2001; Maskovsky 2000; Wacquant

2001; Schneider 1999). Under this neoliberal rubric of responsibility, people needing governmental support are seen as deviant, irresponsible citizens unable to provide for themselves and needing punishment (O'Daniel 2008; Maskovsky 2000). As anthropologists have demonstrated, neoliberalism is more than an economic philosophy; it is also a form of governmentality. As Aihwa Ong argues, neoliberal philosophy involves casting individuals as "living resources that may be harnessed and managed by governing regimes," and whose capacities for capital accumulation, self-governance, efficiency, and productivity must be optimized (2006, 6). Neoliberalism, then, is not only a philosophy of economic intervention but also a way to manage populations.

When understood through a lens of neoliberal governmentality, immigrant policing efforts are an attempt to force self-sufficiency by leveraging fear of apprehension. In other words, immigrant policing efforts operationalize fear to attempt to force immigrants to find their own avenues of care, like the shadow medical system that developed in Atlanta. Thus, immigrant policing regimes reveal ways in which governmental action serves to create a type of ideal neoliberal citizen: one who makes no demands on the state but provides labor, often cheaply. The neoliberal citizen would therefore be a totally harnessable resource made self-sufficient by receiving few benefits, rights, and protections, and controlled through constant reminders of social vulnerability. Such efforts do not always work, however, and immigrants can actively resist immigrant policing regimes, as Palomita demonstrated in refusing to accept police targeting her neighborhood.

Some immigrants' experiences, as I described in this chapter, illustrate how immigrant policing plays a role in creating the "hypercitizen" that anthropologists Heide Castañeda and Milena Melo have described: the citizen who routinely checks a vehicle and drives cautiously to avoid the scrutiny of a harsh immigration regime, embodying a hyperbolic form of cautionary living (Castañeda and Melo 2013). Hypercitizenship practices, like checking vehicles before driving, as Adelina reminded GLAHRiadores to do in the introduction, do not exist in isolation. Instead, they merge with decisions like avoiding certain areas for health care, altering individual health behaviors, and seeking health care from a shadow medical system. Overall, these practices suggest an emerging biopolitics of caution as undocumented immigrants must be overly careful in routine, mundane activities to avoid discovery and potential deportation, and careful in where they seek treatment for illnesses.

Immigrant policing regimes also reveal fundamental contradictions in care for immigrants in Atlanta. Health services for undocumented immigrants are ostensibly available through organizations like CETPA and even large hospitals like Grady, but they are made inaccessible through police activity. Similarly, medications and limited services may be available through a shadow medical system of dubious quality. Overall, the medical landscape in Atlanta consists of several forms of belied care for undocumented immigrants: care that exists but disguises another reality. But belied care is just one way that contradictory social structures exist for some undocumented immigrants, since law enforcement itself has become an entity of belied mission. Whereas police ostensibly exist for public safety and welfare, for undocumented immigrants, police undermine individual safety and wellbeing, and as I describe in the following chapter, destabilize interpersonal relationships.

4 · IMMIGRANT POLICING AND INTERPERSONAL RELATIONSHIPS

Verónica, a tall, thin woman in her mid-twenties, lives in Cartersville, a city of about 20,000 people between Atlanta and Chattanooga, Tennessee. When I met her at her home one morning, Verónica greeted me with a child in her arms, and we sat in her living room talking about her time living in Georgia. Verónica came to the United States in 2000 with her aunt and uncle, and until about five months before we met, before moving to Cartersville, she had lived closer to Atlanta in Cobb County. Like Palomita and her family, Verónica explained that moving was necessary because she was concerned about aggressive immigration enforcement practices.

In her former neighborhood, Verónica had been arrested for driving without a license. "I was coming home from work one day, and a police officer pulled me over," she said. "I wasn't speeding or anything, but he pulled me over and took me to jail for not having a license." The officer failed to give Verónica a valid reason for the stop—after all, he had no way of knowing she lacked a license until he pulled her over. "They let me out of jail, but I learned that I supposedly had an order for my arrest since 2011 from getting stopped at a *retén*." The checkpoint was Verónica's first encounter with law enforcement. "They were checking to see if people were wearing seatbelts, and I was giving a ride to a woman and her kids that weren't wearing seatbelts, so they stopped me, but they didn't take me to jail that day." Verónica thought at the time she was benefiting from the officer's discretion. "The officer was Hispanic and he told me they wouldn't detain us, but he would just give me a ticket. . . . So after that, I got an attorney, and the attorney told me that I didn't have to go to court or anything." Verónica thought the stop and ticket were a benign incident in her past, but she quickly discovered she was wrong. "That [stop] is what I had the order for arrest for, that I didn't know about," she said. Verónica ultimately went to Cobb County jail to serve time for not paying the ticket for the seatbelt infraction. "They let me out," she explained, "but I can't drive or anything because I was told if I got caught again for driving without a license they would take me to immigration. So I don't drive anymore."

Verónica was unsure of why Cobb County police had not handed her over to Immigration and Customs Enforcement (ICE) when she was in jail for the traffic violation, but she did not want to risk additional chances of being apprehended by police. For Verónica, an arrest would mean no one could take care of her three children since her partner, Josue, had been deported to Mexico. "[My children's] father is in Mexico—they deported him. . . . A police officer got him for not having a license; they got him, and immigration got him." Verónica and Josue paid a $7,500 bond for Josue's release from jail, and they waited for him to receive a summons in the mail to appear before an immigration court. ICE made a mistake, however, and never mailed Josue the summons, and he was ultimately arrested and deported. He had been in the United States for nineteen years.

There are several ways in which a person living in the United States can be deported as part of the nation's complex immigration system. If immigrants are in the United States for fewer than fourteen days and apprehended within one hundred miles of a U.S. border, they can be deported immediately in a process known as expedited removal (Gebisa 2007). In many cases, however, the deportation process starts with what I described in chapter 1: When someone like Josue is arrested for driving without a license, they are taken to jail; and under the Secure Communities program, their arrest information is sent to immigration authorities. At that point, ICE can request that local police hold the arrestee for forty-eight hours until agents determine the arrestee's immigration status. Upon determining a lack of authorized status, ICE can issue a notice to appear before an immigration judge and can choose to detain immigrants for indefinite periods of time in detention facilities like the one I describe in chapter 7. If an immigration judge issues an order of removal, ICE ultimately places the detainee on a chartered bus or plane and sends them to their country of birth (Shoichet and Merrill 2017).

The deportation process is complicated and has potential for error. For example, during my time in Atlanta, I met Juan Carlos, a recent high school graduate who came to the United States with his parents when he was an infant. During his senior year in high school, he was driving home from his girlfriend's house in Cobb County, and a drunk driver crashed into his car. He called the police, and when officers arrived, they questioned Juan Carlos's immigration status and arrested him because he did not have a driver's license. After he was arrested, ICE authorities made a procedural error and deported Juan Carlos to Mexico before he appeared in front of an immigration judge. Immigration judges must sign deportation orders, and when his attorneys discovered ICE prematurely deported him without a signed order, immigration authorities returned Juan Carlos to the United States to deport him *again*. The error inspired local activists to request ICE not separate Juan Carlos from his parents, siblings, and high school friends in the community where he grew up, holding press releases and events like one titled "ICE tries to deport Juan Carlos AGAIN!" The events were unsuccessful. Juan Carlos was deported and is currently living in Mexico.[1]

When deported and separated from their families, some immigrants from Latin America will risk their lives and face the consequences of potential apprehension as they attempt to return to the United States. Juan Carlos did not attempt to return, nor did Verónica's former partner, Josue. "He's already married there," Verónica explained. "He says he wants to see his children but I told him I wasn't going to send them because they are too young, and he said he thinks he can see them later, but who knows. We talk on the phone so at least he can talk to his children, but who knows if he'll ever get to see them again." As Verónica and Josue's situation suggests, family separation is a common aspect of immigrant policing.

Verónica fears that, like Josue, she could be arrested, deported, and separated from her children. She tried to apply for temporary relief from deportation granted through the Deferred Action for Childhood Arrivals (DACA) so that she could avoid being deported, but she had difficulty with completing the requirements of the application. DACA provides a temporary reprieve from deportation and allows undocumented immigrants to obtain work permits if they meet certain eligibility criteria. To be eligible, applicants must have entered the United States before age sixteen, must have lived in the United States continuously since 2007, must have completed or be pursuing a high school degree or its equivalent, must not have committed any crimes, and must be younger than thirty-one years old at the time of application. Applicants must also pay a fee of nearly $500 for their application and provide proof of their residency and work history. For immigrants like Verónica, who was paid in cash with no formal agreement with an employer, employment history can be hard to come by. When Verónica consulted an attorney about applying for DACA, she had trouble collecting all the requisite documents. "They ask for proof that I got here when I was 14 and I don't really have proof because I worked in restaurants and they paid me in cash, so I'm going to see if one restaurant owner will write me a letter, but I haven't found him. And they ask that you enroll in school, but I'm looking for a school close to here because I don't want to drive."

When the Obama administration created DACA in 2012, the program responded to ongoing congressional and political debates about immigration reform that focused on undocumented youth as a desirable class of "potential citizens" born to parents who brought them to the United States. DACA is not citizenship, and because of its temporary nature it is in a constant state of flux. In 2017, the Trump administration ended the program, but successful legal challenges required the administration to keep the program indefinitely; however, congressional action could potentially end DACA. At the time of writing this book, the future of DACA is uncertain, and not all immigrants, like Verónica, can benefit from it.

Because Verónica does not drive, she relies on her boyfriend, Antonio, for transportation. Antonio has a valid driver's license from another state that he shows if he gets pulled over. "One time they pulled Antonio over and asked for his license, and he showed it to the police and the officer said 'okay, well if you're going to live here you have to get a license here.'" But as Verónica noted, she and Antonio were undocumented and were not eligible for a Georgia driver's license. "They don't give us [licenses] here! They don't want us to have a license!" Without a license, and when Antonio is at work, Verónica is confined to her house. Like Martina, she described not being able to leave her house as much as she would like to. "You stay put," she explained. "[It is] difficult—you're unable to work and unable to do anything. You can't safely go out into the street because you think they're going to pull you over." Being unable to drive not only limits where Verónica can go but also restricts what she feels she can do for her children. "I have children who have appointments, so I can't get to the pediatrician or the dentist either." Verónica asks friends for rides to appointments for her children; there is no public transportation where she lives. "There's no bus here," she explained.

Verónica's children were born in the United States and are U.S. citizens; because of their citizenship, they are eligible for Medicaid. Despite their eligibility, Verónica refused to accept benefits for her children until shortly before we met, and only then because she desperately needed the financial assistance in caring for them. "I didn't want to get Medicaid for them because their father was making good money, but right now, as I said, I'm all alone. . . . The father of my children was deported." Verónica's refusal to accept social services for her children counters narratives about immigrants being "drains" on social services. Her U.S.-citizen children are eligible for and entitled to publicly funded programs like Medicaid, but Verónica avoided using services for them when she felt she had sufficient finances to pay out of pocket for their needs. This refusal also reflects how undocumented immigrants may avoid using public services as a way of not "being a public charge" (Horton 2014).

When I asked Verónica how she felt about the challenges in taking care of children and being unable to drive, she began to cry. "I just feel so much despair because I have no job and I have my children I have to look after." Although Verónica has a boyfriend who provides for her economically, she explained feeling guilty for not being able to work. "My boyfriend helps me sometimes but it's a big burden for him, paying for the house, the car insurance, the bills, and everything. It's really hard for him by himself, and I want to work, I tell him 'I'm going to have to work,' but he says 'no,' he expects me not to drive, but you need to drive because you need to work. Sometimes it's just so frustrating that you can't—." Verónica, overwhelmed with tears, was unable to finish her sentence. "I have to care for my children," she said, pausing for a moment, and wiping the tears streaming down her face.

Verónica's situation highlights a number of ways in which immigrant policing affects interpersonal relationships and magnifies gendered expectations of care and domestic responsibility. Although Verónica's boyfriend financially assisted her, economic dependence in some immigrant families may create or contribute to unhealthy and potentially harmful relationships. Economic challenges play a key role in intimate partner violence, and economic dependence on a partner is one of several factors that may be present in abusive relationships (Bornstein 2006).

In this chapter, I describe how immigrant policing can disrupt interpersonal relationships, focusing primarily on parent-child relationships and intimate partnerships. I show how immigrant policing destabilizes interpersonal relationships by creating persistent threats of family separation and producing stressors that contribute to intimate partner violence. These interpersonal consequences have directly informed activist efforts to challenge oppressive immigration enforcement regimes, but as I will show, such efforts typically focus on heterosexual families with children, ignoring other types of relationships, like same-sex couples or couples without children. In addressing these topics, I show how fear as a biopolitical technology of control modifies some immigrants' interpersonal relationships and exacerbates gender-related vulnerabilities and inequalities. I should note that although immigrant policing can disrupt a number of interpersonal and family relationships—including those between siblings, adults and elderly parents, intimate partners without legally recognized relationships, and others—in this chapter I focus significantly on heterosexual nuclear families with children. These families were ones I got to know through GLAHR and other organizations, but they do not account for the full extent to which immigrant policing unsettles relationships between individuals.

CHILDREN AND IMMIGRANT POLICING

In 2018, the Trump administration announced a "zero tolerance policy" for immigrants and their families crossing into the United States from the U.S.-Mexico border (Department of Homeland Security 2018). As part of the policy, parents were sent to federal prisons and separated from their children, who were placed in shelters operated by the Department of Health and Human Services (HHS). At the time of writing this book, more than 14,000 children were held in the HHS shelters, putting the facilities at their capacity (Moghe and Flores 2018) and resulting in the Trump administration converting a defunct Walmart store into a child detention center and creating a makeshift "tent city" facility for migrant children (Fernandez 2018). The stressful and traumatic circumstances surrounding parent-child separation raised concerns among medical professionals, who warned the administration that the toxic stress resulting from separation could hinder brain development and result in long-term adverse health consequences (K. Phillips 2018; J. Rose 2018). News media reported that the administration deported some parents without their children, made no attempt to reunite separated families in some cases, and intentionally designed the zero tolerance policy to discourage immigrants from entering the United States by making them fearful of losing family members (Carrasquero 2018; Kopan 2018). Just as immigrant policing tactics used fear as a biopolitical technology of control that altered immigrants' health-related behavior, as I described in the previous chapter, the zero tolerance policy leveraged families as a biopolitical exercise. Such an effort is not exclusive to the border or to the zero tolerance policy, however. On the contrary, the immigrant policing regimes I have described throughout this book have resulted in family separation and used fear as a technology of control, but arguably in a more covert manner.

An estimated 4.5–5.5 million children in the United States have at least one undocumented parent, and the majority of those children (4.1 million) are U.S. citizens (Zayas and Bradlee 2014; Dreby 2012a, 2012b). In families where both parents are in the United States, when one parent is deported, children will typically remain with the other parent (see, for example, Dreby 2012a). When both parents are deported, children may stay with relatives or return with their parents, but in some cases, children of undocumented immigrants can be placed with foster parents. States can terminate undocumented immigrants' parental rights (Zayas and Bradlee 2014; Andrapalliyal 2013), and as a result, more than 5,000 children in the U.S. foster care system are children of deported parents (Human Impact Partners 2013). In Georgia, an official I met with from the Department of Family and Children Services (DFCS) explained that undocumented status was sometimes a problematic factor in considering parents' rights to stay with children. "Sometimes you see that being undocumented is considered against the parent— it's a liability, and the state will see that it's not in the best interest of [the] child to be with an undocumented parent, so they put the children with foster parents." Although DFCS officials have claimed documentation status is not a factor in determining whether parents maintain custody of their children, news reports highlighted at least one high-profile incident in which DFCS allegedly refused to reunite Latinx parents with their children because of the parents' documentation status and language ability (Trevizo 2011; Wessler 2011).

Through separating children and parents, immigration policies directly impact children dependent on parents by creating "two classes of vulnerable citizen-children: exiles . . . and orphans" (Zayas and Bradlee 2014, 169). Exiles are children who leave the United States with their parents, and orphans are those who are left in the United States and cared for by others, including the child welfare system (Zayas and Bradlee 2014). Despite its association with detrimental emotional and economic impacts on children across their life course (Zayas and

Bradlee 2014; Chaudry et al. 2010; Barajas, Philipsen, and Brooks-Gunn 2008; Leventhal and Brooks-Gunn 2004), parent-child separation continues through immigrant policing regimes.

In addition to young children and parents being separated, adult children who came to the United States with their parents can be deported and leave behind families in which there are several different types of immigration statuses, such as undocumented parents and U.S. citizen siblings. This is what happened to Juan Carlos after ICE, as he explained to me, "brought [him] back to the country to be deported again the right way." Beyond the absurdity of being deported and returned to the United States only to be deported again, Juan Carlos's experience reveals how undocumented young adults who arrived in the United States as children can find themselves in situations in which they are simultaneously exiled and orphaned.

Many immigrants I met in Atlanta described concerns about being deported and possibly separated from their children. Several also discussed the economic hardships resulting from spousal deportation. One woman, Estrella, explained: "My husband was deported and now I have to care for my children by myself. I don't work or drive because there are police." For Estrella, her children's separation from their father felt deeply unjust: "They deserve to have their father here with them. They're from this country and they deserve to grow up with their father," she tearfully asserted. Although she found assistance with rent and bills through her church, Estrella was unsure how she would continue to support herself over a longer period of time. "I need to be here for my children," she explained.

Stories like Verónica's and Estrella's were commonly discussed in *comité popular* meetings and were used as part of GLAHR's immigrant policing resistance narrative. Acting on concerns of family separation, GLAHR organized political actions around the topic, including a political bus tour to legislators' offices titled "Keeping Families Together," and several *teatro popular* (popular theater) events (figure 7). Teatro popular is a type of "theatre of the oppressed," which uses theater to build social networks, draw attention to social injustices, and share strategies for overcoming various forms of oppression (Wernick, Kulick, and Woodford 2014; Faigin and Stein 2010; Howard 2004; Sanders 2004; Boal 2000). One of the GLAHRiadores, Alfonso, led the teatro popular endeavors, which were usually performed at the Plaza Fiesta shopping mall on a weekend. These events featured educational components and calls for political action, as demonstrated by the first performance I participated in. In this performance, I played the role of George W. Bush, speaking Spanish in an exaggerated southern U.S. accent through a mask of the former president (figure 8). One of the goals of the performance was to inform the local community about the history and genesis of immigration laws. The plot of the performance included a child's parent being arrested while driving, highlighting how policies passed during the Bush administration,

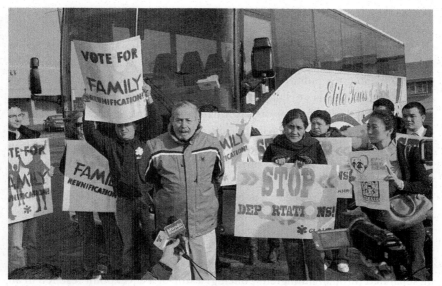

FIGURE 7. The start of the "Keeping Families Together" bus tour. (Photo by Ponciano Ugalde.)

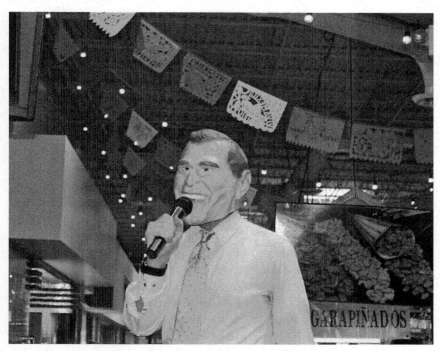

FIGURE 8. When anthropologists act: playing George W. Bush in a teatro popular. (Photo by Ponciano Ugalde.)

like the REAL ID Act (which I described in chapter 1), culminated in real-world impacts that affected immigrant children.

In addition to educating audiences, teatro popular events aimed to spark action among viewers. By tying together the real daily hardships immigrants face with education about the political history leading to those hardships, teatro popular events directed viewers to take action, including writing letters to Congress or joining GLAHR. The merger of performance, education, and calls for political action was perhaps best demonstrated during the second teatro popular I participated in. In this performance, I played the role of a young boy in elementary school whose friend María did not show up for school that day. As the teatro unfolded, audience members learned that María had not come to school because her father had been stopped by a police officer and arrested for driving without a license. At the end of the ten-minute-long teatro, audience members were asked to write to Congress to stop deportations, with the help of GLAHRiadores who supplied pens and paper.

These performances highlighted to audiences how immigrant families could be separated through immigrant policing: a stop at a checkpoint resulted in an arrest for driving without a license, which led to an ICE hold and eventual detention and deportation made possible through a local jail in a Secure Communities jurisdiction. The teatros were more than just performance, however, as the "actors" were performing scenarios they could encounter at any point in their lives. This was made especially clear to me during one of our rehearsals for the teatro involving the story of María. At the rehearsal, Adelina asked the GLAHRiadores if they had a plan for their children in case they were arrested (figures 9 and 10).

"We've talked to [our daughter]," one GLAHRiador said, "but nothing is written." Adelina stressed to everyone in the room why they must have written plans. "It's very important you have these things in writing. What if you and your wife are both arrested, what happens to your children?" Mari, a GLAHRiador, responded, and explained that she and her husband, Felipe, have written instructions for who should care for their five-year-old daughter, Alexis, if they are both deported. "Alexis knows that if we don't come home where she should go," Mari said. "She knows where to find the papers that say who she should stay with if we get sent back." Adelina nodded. "It's very important to do this if you haven't already," she added. "Who do you want making decisions about your children? You, or some lawyer?" One GLAHRiador called to Alexis. "Alexis, do you know where to go if something happens to your parents?" Looking to Alexis, Mari restated the question. "Who do you stay with if your father and I don't come home?" Eyes wide and maintaining her nearly always-present grin, Alexis responded "mi tía Gloria!" Mari hugged Alexis. "That's right!" Mari exclaimed.

For Mari, Felipe, and Alexis, the potential of family separation through deportation was more than a teatro performance. Instead, it was a constant pos-

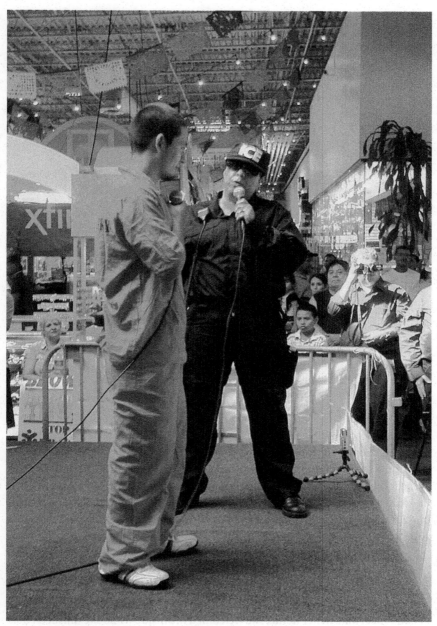

FIGURE 9. A scene in the first teatro popular. (Photo by Nolan Kline.)

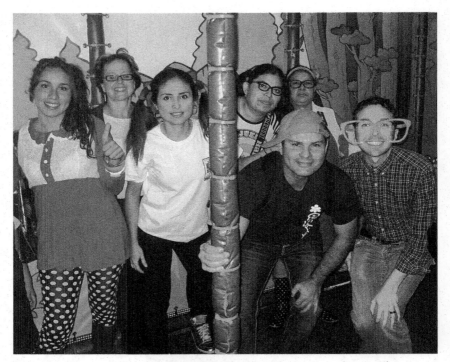

FIGURE 10. The cast of the second teatro popular featuring the story of María. The anthropologist Martha Rees, an Atlanta resident who has worked with GLAHR, is second from the left. (Photo by Ponciano Ugalde.)

sibility that required planning. Mari, Felipe, and Alexis had talked about potential plans of care if Mari and Felipe were apprehended by police or deported. In addition to the copies of their plans in their home for family and law enforcement to find if necessary, they also had copies of this paperwork with Alexis's *tía* (aunt). Mari and Felipe were not unusual in their preparations; other undocumented immigrants I met in Atlanta, like Anita, a mother of four, made similar plans.

CONTINGENCY PLANS, GENDERED EXPECTATIONS, AND INTERSECTIONALITY

When I met Anita in her home, she welcomed me inside while she finished cooking a meal. "*Siéntate, por favor,*" she said, ushering me into her kitchen and gesturing to the table. "Go set the other table," Anita instructed one of her daughters, who then brought a folding table out from another room and covered it with a white tablecloth. A few minutes later, Anita began serving plates of rice and beans with tortillas, grilled pork, and vegetables. As we sat and ate at a small table by the kitchen, Anita's four children—the youngest twelve, the oldest twenty-two—ate next to us at the other table.

Anita arrived in the United States in 1999 with her husband, Carlos, and three of her children. She initially worked a variety of hospitality jobs, including working in a posh hotel in downtown Atlanta, housed in one of the city's iconic high-rises. When she and Carlos arrived in the United States, Carlos got a driver's license, but he was unable to renew it when it expired because of changes made to Georgia law that excluded undocumented immigrants from receiving licenses. With 287(g), Secure Communities, and HB 87 resulting in immigrants being arrested and deported, Carlos feared leaving the house.

"He started to panic," Anita explained. "He didn't want to drive anymore." Anita told Carlos that they had to drive and continue working. "We're here, we have to go out. And he said 'the police are here in front of our house, it's possible they're going to pull you over.' And I told him we have to drive, we have to leave to go to work, we have to leave to get food for the children." Anita and Carlos disagreed about whether to stay in the United States, and Carlos ultimately decided to return to Mexico on his own in December 2011 because he feared getting arrested by police and held in detention for an unpredictable amount of time.

Without Carlos in Atlanta, Anita described that she alone bore the responsibility for her and her children's survival; and when we met, she routinely drove to work. Anita recognized the risks in driving and was unsure of what would happen to her every time she left the house. "Every day I leave for work, but I don't know if I'll return." Anita fears what may happen to her children if she is deported. "What will my children do without me? I remember a time I got sick and went to the hospital and my children didn't eat because Carlos didn't know what to make and didn't take them to a restaurant. They didn't eat! I was in the hospital for three or four days because I had a seizure."

Anita's situation underscores how many women in the United States shoulder the burden for child care and household economics alone, and further exemplifies how women increasingly have been engaged in transnational labor migration since the 1990s (Horton 2009). Some specific types of labor have reinforced gendered notions of women as caregivers responsible for domestic affairs. For example, Latinx women in certain parts of the United States play a vital role in caring for U.S. citizens' children as domestic employees (Hondagneu-Sotelo 2001), revealing a deep irony in labor and immigration enforcement patterns that can result in domestic care workers potentially being separated from their own children on their way to work and care for someone else's. Thousands of U.S. citizen parents depend on Latinx women for child care and other domestic labor. The growing demand for women working in the service sector, and the emergence of intensified immigration enforcement regimes has, as Sarah Horton writes, "paved the way for increased deportation and family separation" (2009, 24), amplifying gender-related labor expectations in and outside the home.

After Anita's husband returned to Mexico and she alone had to meet the economic needs of her household, she felt a heightened necessity to sacrifice personal needs in order to care for her family. She explained that she cannot allow herself to become ill or be caught driving without a license because any type of downtime could harm her family. "I can't get sick and I can't get stopped by police—what are my children going to do? If anything happens to me it's my children I'm most worried about. And they're always telling me 'don't work so much, eat well, don't get sick!'" Anytime she gets behind the wheel of her car, Anita prays to not be pulled over and taken from her family.

Anthropologists have described how family separation disrupts parent-child bonds and results in numerous types of distress (Horton 2009, 22–23). U.S. policy is the root cause of these disruptions, and as anthropologist Deborah Boehm (2012) argues, the U.S. state directly impacts migrants' familial relationships and gendered expectations about such relationships. Boehm (2012, 81) shows how in households where men and women are separated, women take on roles previously performed by men, and some explain that they "do everything." Transnational movement therefore results in frequently shifting gender roles (Boehm 2012, 89), as in Anita's household. Before Carlos's return to Mexico, Anita was the primary caregiver for her children but shared the economic burden of providing for their household with Carlos. After he left, Anita was the only caretaker for her children and was solely responsible for household economic stability.

The ways in which immigrant policing results in gender shifts underscore how intersecting identities as a racial minority, woman, and someone without papers merge to create distinct lived experiences for women like Anita. As legal scholar Kimberlé Crenshaw (1989) has argued, forms of discrimination based on social phenomena like sex or race do not operate independently of one another. Instead, multiple forms of discrimination that some populations encounter intersect and create qualitatively unique forms of disenfranchisement (Crenshaw 1989, 140). Crenshaw's concept of intersectionality underscores how layered forms of social subordination like sex and race create new subjectivities. For example, black women in the United States encounter sexism that black men do not, and experience racism that white women do not. For undocumented women like Anita, sex, gender, and documentation status intersect in ways that shape their lived experiences.

Like Anita, other undocumented interviewees expressed concern about what would happen to their children if they were deported, and they prepared for such possibilities. Silvia, for example, a mother with two children, explained, "I say goodbye to my children every time I leave the house because I know I may not see them again." The threat of family separation led Silvia, like Mari and Felipe, to prepare instructions for her children if she were arrested. "See that table over there?" Silvia said to me while we sat in her home, gesturing to a small console table with drawers. "There's a folder in there with instructions for where to go and who to contact if I don't come home. My daughter knows that if I don't come home that she should take that folder and go to the neighbor's house."

These preparations for children demonstrate the importance of social support in the context of immigrant policing. As public health scholars have shown, social support includes both being integrated in a social network and having access to emotional and instrumental assistance (see, for example, Reblin and Uchino 2008). As some undocumented families must rely on friends and other family members to care for their children in case of being detained or deported, social support is a critical way to mitigate the consequences of intense immigrant policing.

Although some parents prepared for possible family separation, preparedness did not necessarily alleviate anxieties over family separation, particularly among children. As a children's mental health provider at one organization explained, "Children are so anxious and so afraid their parents are going to get deported that they're afraid to get in the car. I see kids drawing pictures of their dads getting arrested, and kids aren't doing as well in school because they're anxious and worried about what's going to happen to their mom or to their dad while they're in school." While adults experience anxiety and trauma when encountering a police car, as I described in the previous chapter, their children also fear what might happen if their parents have such an encounter.

Sofia, a leader of a family services organization that serves Latinx men, women, and children, explained how fear related to immigrant policing resulted in anxiety among children who come to her organization. "With the younger kids we see a lot of reporting of the headaches and stomachaches, a lot of the physical stuff, which is the way that they're internalizing some of the anxiety and the fear." Sofia added that fear led some children to not want to leave their parents during the day: "We've had kids who are afraid to go to school because they're afraid their parents might not be there by the time they get back. For a lot of families when they get pulled over, it wasn't at 3 o'clock in the morning, it was on the way to the grocery store [getting stopped] for an imaginary taillight that went out." Sofia explained how some immigrant children may blame themselves for their parents' arrests and deportations. "I know one youth in particular who blames herself because her mom got pulled over after she asked her mom to take her to the grocery store to pick out a birthday cake for her brother, or her dad, or somebody, and her mom got pulled over on the way to the grocery store with her daughter, and long story short, the mom ended up getting deported."

According to Sofia, the sense of blame translated to this girl attempting to replace her mother because she felt responsible for her deportation. "So this child ended up dropping out of school to help take care of family and kind of replace the mom and her role. She blamed herself for asking for the cake and she thinks she caused it. It's just sad because it wasn't her fault, but you saw the impact on her life and now she is trying to get a GED [a type of certification for completing high-school level skills]." Anxieties about police do not stop as children age into

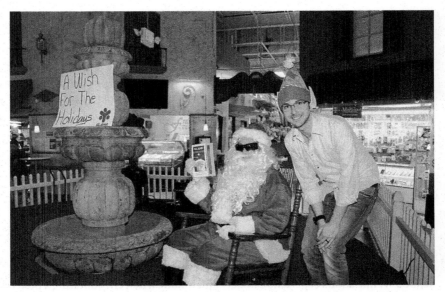

FIGURE 11. Playing Santa's elf during a GLAHR letter-writing action. (Photo by Ponciano Ugalde.)

adults: "It's just frustrating at times to see this all happening—the kids are suffering and they keep suffering when they're adults," Sofia exclaimed. As I described in the previous chapter, immigrant policing results in internalizing policies through expressing fear. Children may also live with the constant fear some immigrants described, potentially increasing long-term depression and anxiety and creating negative consequences that last across the life course.

In response to children and parents fearing being separated from one another, GLAHR organized events to encourage adults and children to take political action. At a December event, titled "A Wish for the Holidays" (figure 11), GLAHR staff and I helped children write letters to Congress to request that ICE agents end deportations so that children could spend the holidays with their parents. By the end of the event, we had collected nearly seventy letters, which GLAHR staff mailed to individual members of Congress along with other letters and pictures from GLAHRiadores' children. Overall, the Wish for the Holidays letter-writing action and the teatros demonstrate how GLAHR and its members actively resisted the kinds of pressures immigrant policing placed on immigrants' parent and child relationships. Rather than accepting deportation and parent-child separation as inevitable, GLAHRiadores took political action to demand policy changes. Using a family lens to appeal to legislators may allow for an emotionally driven type of activism that can potentially sway policy makers and combat ways in which immigrant policing intervenes in interpersonal relationships. But parent-child separation is not the only example of how immigrant policing can alter interpersonal relationships.

ACTIVISM AND DATING WHILE UNDOCUQUEER

As I discovered in the fieldwork resulting in this book, immigrant policing complicated interpersonal relationships for undocumented lesbian, gay, bisexual, transgender, and otherwise queer-identifying (LGBTQ+) immigrants. At a gay bar in midtown Atlanta near a strip mall known as the heart of Atlanta's "gayborhood," I sat outside with Sammy and Hiran, who came to Atlanta on the undocubus—a brightly painted bus they named Priscilla after the film *Priscilla, Queen of the Desert*. As members of the "No Papers, No Fear Ride for Justice" demonstration, Sammy and Hiran joined other undocumented immigrants traveling across the southern U.S. states to raise awareness about immigrant policing, build resistance to anti-immigrant laws, and ultimately have their voices heard at the 2012 Democratic National Convention. When we met, I had been dressed for my role as George W. Bush in the teatro, and Sammy thought I was a lawyer: "We all thought you were the lawyer," he laughed. "Usually if there's someone dressed like you [were for the teatro] then they're the lawyer. Every one of these groups has a lawyer and it's usually the only white person in the room." In a quieter section of the bar's outdoor courtyard, Hiran described frustration with being a gay man on an immigrant rights tour across the U.S. South. When driving to a church hosting the bus in a rural Georgia town, for example, Hiran explained that the bus driver got a call from church leadership requesting that no one talk about anything related to identifying as LGBTQ+. The request upset Hiran; he identifies as both gay and undocumented, or "undocuqueer," and being asked to closet himself in a church was hurtful. He understood the request, however, since the church was not welcoming to LGBTQ+ people, but this created a unique problem. Although the church welcomed undocumented immigrants, it would not accept someone who identified as gay. This form of exclusion is only one part of the type of exclusion he and other undocuqueer men and women regularly experience.

For men like Hiran and Sammy, being undocumented and LGBTQ+ are equally important aspects of their identities. Sometimes being both undocumented and gay results in undocuqueer individuals having multiple coming-out processes, each with its associated challenges. Coming out as gay, for example, can be complicated in spaces that welcome undocumented immigrants, such as the church where Hiran and Sammy stayed in rural Georgia. Similarly, coming out as undocumented to a romantic or sexual partner can be difficult and end relationships. As Hiran explained, "I've had guys not see me anymore once I tell them I'm undocumented." In other cases, more understanding partners are uninformed about how Hiran and Sammy are undocumented. "Guys I've been with say 'why don't you just go down to the courthouse and fix it?' But they don't get it—it's not that simple," Hiran explained. Indeed, as anthropologist Ruth Gomberg-Muñoz (2016) has written, "fixing" immigration status is not simple, and in the case of intimate partner relationships like spouses, adjusting an immigration status can result in couples being apart for a decade or ultimately having to dissolve their relationship[2].

Immigrant policing directly influenced the layered or multiple closets that Hiran and Sammy found themselves in as undocuqueer men. At their church, they could freely talk about their immigration status and not worry about judgment, but the two men could not talk about being gay. Conversely, at the gay bar where we sat outside while drag queens performed inside, Hiran and Sammy could talk about being gay without judgment, but felt they could not disclose their immigration status there. They did not frequently find spaces where they could discuss being both undocumented *and* gay. Additionally, in some situations, immigrant policing efforts directly complicated their ability to get into LGBTQ+ spaces where they could meet potential partners. More specifically, getting into a gay bar or club at all was complicated because of their immigration status. "We don't have driver's licenses, so if they're checking IDs and won't accept a passport, we can't get in," Sammy noted.

As Hiran and Sammy's experiences reveal, immigrant policing can directly impact undocuqueer immigrants' relationships and hinder their ability to retreat to social spaces designed to be safe for LGBTQ+ people, such as gay bars. Moreover, their experiences reveal the intersecting vulnerabilities of being undocumented and a sexual minority. Just as immigrant policing efforts uniquely alter undocumented women's lives in unique ways, they also contribute to distinct challenges in undocuqueer men's interpersonal relationships. When put into context with activist appeals focused on children and one male and one female parent, Hiran and Sammy's experiences also underscore the limits of activist efforts focused on heterosexual families and families with children. These efforts can problematically reinforce romanticized, gendered, heteronormative notions of families that also reinforce divisions between citizens and noncitizens (Heidbrink 2014, 2; Pallares 2014; Zavella 2012, 1).

Because immigrant policing alters interpersonal relationships and has the potential to reproduce gendered, heterosexist forms of activism, immigration enforcement efforts serve as a way to reinforce divisions between LGBTQ+ and non-LGBTQ+ men and women. Immigrant policing creates figurative borders between communities that could be united in their resistance to xenophobia, racism, homophobia, sexism, and other forms of hatred. The church where Hiran and Sammy were told they could not express themselves could have more effectively combated the divisions immigrant policing creates by welcoming *all* immigrants, not just those who identify as straight.

The types of challenges Hiran and Sammy described in finding romantic partners also shed light on how immigrant policing can structure intimate partner relationships through creating metaphorical walls between people. Gay men who dump Hiran or Sammy because of their immigration status participate in the continual division of groups, particularly among LGBTQ+ groups. Such divisions are not exclusive to citizenship status but also include race, body shape and type, and other features and characteristics. Combined, the manner in which immigrant policing impacts interpersonal relationships among undocuqueer men, and between children and parents, demonstrates how immigration enforcement efforts are a power technique that can pervade numerous settings and interact with other techniques of power designed to govern populations, like race, gender, and sexual orientation. This became clear to me as I examined how immigrant policing could impact intimate partner relationships by exacerbating existing or potential intimate partner violence and impeding intervention efforts.

FEAR, POLICE, AND INTERPERSONAL VIOLENCE

During one of the weekly comité popular meetings Doña Julia led, I tried to arrange an interview with Leticia, a woman with a teenage daughter and young son. Leticia lived across the parking lot from Doña Julia and frequently went to meetings.

"You should talk to Nolan," Julia insisted one evening, as we all stood in the parking lot outside the apartment complex's basketball courts where we met by a group of picnic tables. "He is learning about all the hardships we face—all the checkpoints and people being arrested, all the families being broken up. You should talk to him!"

Julia had been trying to help me arrange an interview with Leticia for several weeks, and Leticia typically had reasons for why she could not participate in an interview, such as not knowing a good time to talk. That evening, Leticia looked anxious when Julia insisted she speak with me.

"My husband doesn't really like people coming over," Leticia explained.

"Your husband?" Julia asked. "It's okay, Nolan will just talk to *you*."

I began to feel that Leticia was being coerced and wanted to find a way out of the situation: "It's okay, if you don't want to, you don't have to! I'm really hungry anyway, so I need to head out and grab dinner."

Julia turned to me. "Leticia can make you pizza," she said. "Nolan likes pizza," Julia said, turning back to Leticia. "You should talk to him. He's recording the story of what's happening to our community."

"I just need to talk to my husband first," Leticia said with a concerned expression.

"It's okay, I have to go anyway," I insisted.

"Okay, talk to your husband and then next week you can talk to Nolan," Julia said definitively.

"Okay, next week if my husband says it's okay," Leticia responded.

"Yes, next week, and you can have pizza," Julia confirmed, with a decisive nod to me. The comité met the following week, and after the meeting I followed Leticia to her apartment. She seemed anxious, and I assumed she was not yet comfortable with me.

"You really don't have to talk to me if you don't want to," I said, as we walked across the parking lot of the apartment complex.

"No, it's okay, and like Julia says, it's helping our community. Someone should know what we go through." I followed Leticia into a quiet, dimly lit apartment where she instructed me to sit at her dining table and disappeared into the kitchen. From the table, I could see her two children staring at the small television from which most of the light filling the space emanated.

"You like pizza?" She asked, peering from behind the doorway that led into the small galley kitchen, breaking the uncanny silence that persisted even as her children watched television.

"Yes, but you don't need to make anything—I'm okay," I answered, getting up to see if I could help with anything.

"It's okay," Leticia responded, taking a packaged pizza out of her freezer and heating her oven. "Go sit." I returned to my seat and heard pieces of cardboard separating from one another and a frozen pizza being placed onto a baking rack with a thud. Leticia returned to the table where she sat across from me. I placed a voice recorder in front of her, and as we began the interview, Leticia's children started playing a game. Their laughter disrupted a dog I had not noticed until I heard a bark from what I had thought was an empty dog carrier against the wall.

"Shhhhhh," Leticia whimpered, frowning at her children. As the dog continued to respond to the children's noise, Leticia opened the carrier and repeatedly told her children to be quiet even though the noise level was hardly disruptive to our interview.

"It's okay—this recorder will still pick up what you say," I explained. Leticia looked at me with a confused expression.

"The noise is okay—they don't have to be quiet," I assured her. As we continued our interview, Leticia interrupted her children's game and had her youngest child, who had been laughing while playing with his sibling, join us. He sat on her lap, restlessly climbing over Leticia, taking periodic breaks to stare into the room, fidgeting. He was bored and wanted to resume playing. Not long after Leticia placed her son on her lap, a man appeared from the hallway leading to the bedrooms and bathroom. As he appeared at the threshold of the doorway, he stood in silence and scowled. Leticia looked at him as he looked at me, and I stood up and introduced myself.

"I'm Nolan, a volunteer with GLAHR," I said, extending my hand.

"Manuel," the man answered, shaking my hand and looking over at Leticia.

"I've got him being quiet now," Leticia said. Manuel nodded, and disappeared into the dark hallway.

"My husband," Leticia said. Suddenly our interview had an entirely new meaning to me. I no longer felt responsible for the heavy air and awkward feeling I had in the silent, dark apartment. Although I had no evidence for my intuition, I sensed Leticia was afraid of more than the police, and as she told me that only her husband left the house and she seldom did, I began to feel her relationship with Manuel was not positive. After we ended our interview, and I left her apartment confused about her home life, I began wondering whether Doña Julia and others in the comité suspected anything about Leticia's relationship. Several weeks after we spoke, Leticia arrived at a comité meeting with a bruise on her face, which she attributed to her son accidentally hitting her in the eye. I became more concerned that Leticia was experiencing physical violence at home. This led me to seek out intimate partner violence (IPV) organizations so that I could provide information to anyone I suspected may need it, and to further consider how IPV and immigrant policing may be related.

IPV is any type of violence against a current or previous spouse, boyfriend, or girlfriend, regardless of gender or sexual orientation, resulting in physical, sexual, or psychological harm (Modi, Palmer, and Armstrong 2014; Bostock, Plumpton, and Pratt 2009; Greenwood et al. 2002; West 2002; Tjaden and Thoennes 2000). It is associated with substantial economic and health-related burdens, including death, injury, disability, chronic illness, and poor mental health (Modi, Palmer, and Armstrong 2014; Wong and Mellor 2014; Ellsberg et al. 2008; Plichta 2004). Among immigrants, violence may increase after immigrating to the United States (Tjaden and Thoennes 2000), and conditions related to immigration may exacerbate existing violence (Menjívar and Salcido 2002). Many immigrants may not report violence to authorities because they fear having their immigration status discovered (Raj et al. 2004), and linguistic, economic, and social barriers may increasingly isolate immigrants experiencing IPV and contribute to not knowing where to receive appropriate services (Modi, Palmer, and Armstrong 2014). For undocumented immigrants in particular, IPV is complicated by issues surrounding legal status, particularly in mixed legal status relationships (Parson et al. 2016). Some partners use immigration status fears as methods of control and violence (Parson et al. 2016; Erez, Adelman, and Gregory 2008; Salcido and Adelman 2004; Abraham 2000). Despite federal legislation for addressing IPV, existing legal protections inadequately address the needs of immigrants at risk for or already experiencing IPV.[3]

In searching for resources for Leticia, I found two organizations that provide IPV services to undocumented immigrants: the Partnership Against Domestic Violence (PADV) and Caminar Latino. PADV provides housing, legal advocacy, a crisis hotline, and various community outreach services; and Caminar Latino focuses on support group and intervention services. Caminar Latino also includes a household-based approach to preventing violence from continuing in the home, and targets partners and children. Caminar Latino counselors and group facilitators meet with entire families and separate men, women, and children into support groups and counseling sessions. At these groups, anyone in the family can share their perspectives about household violence. It was through Caminar Latino that I met Sofia, who provided insight about children fearing their parents' deportation.

Although Caminar Latino serves women, men, and children, most of the organization's clients are adult women. Annually, Caminar Latino serves 400–500 women, fifty men, and 200–250 children, with participating children divided into groups based on age. One of the groups, which comprises high school–aged children, conducted an ethnographic study on the impact of immigrant policing on their families and presented their findings at national conferences. I heard first-hand from the high school students who worked on the report and presented their experiences in feeling targeted by police when I joined a group discussion during one of Caminar Latino's group nights. The students shared that they felt immigration laws were racist policies and heightened household stressors leading to violence. They felt immigrant policing made their parents more frustrated and more likely to fight. Specifically, the students explained that policing worsened the family's financial circumstances because the presence of police meant their parents avoided roadways and had greater difficulty finding work, and the resulting financial tension sometimes led to violent arguments.

Immigration itself plays a role in experiencing and reporting violence. Immigrants may be isolated from friends and family who provide needed social support, may have language challenges that shape employment opportunities, may experience difficulties adapting to a new environment, and may be susceptible to coercion related to their legal status (Menjívar and Salcido 2002). Immigrant policing efforts can heighten these factors since the presence of police in local neighborhoods, as Martina described in the previous chapter, can serve as an immediate reminder of immigrants' vulnerability and deportability. Immigrant policing may also ultimately alter some intimate partner relationships and can be a unique factor that shapes some immigrants' households. In the following section, I focus on immigrant women's experiences of violence in heterosexual relationships because these were the scenarios service providers discussed with me, but this is not meant to ignore men's experiences of violence or violence that occurs in nonheterosexual relationships.

COERCION, TRANSNATIONAL THREATS, AND SEXUAL VIOLENCE

Marta, a victim advocate at a local IPV organization, left an abusive husband in Mexico to find work in the United States. "It got so bad I had no choice but to leave the country with my kids," Marta explained. She has lived in Atlanta for over a decade and became a lawful permanent resident after marrying her second husband. At the IPV organization where she works, Marta helps clients navigate the U.S. legal system and provides them with emotional support. "I went through what they're going through and I know how they feel; I know from experience."

During one of our conversations, Marta noted that for many of her clients, social networks can contribute to coercive relationships. Although being part of a social network can increase social support needed for crafting care-related contingency plans for children and finding safe spaces in violent relationships, Marta explained that this could also contribute to unique forms of vulnerability among some immigrant women. "When [immigrants] move here they move into the same communities [as one another], and they are so isolated because of language and everybody's going to the same place, the same church, and everybody knows each other." A small social network can cause concern when some immigrants worry about reporting violence, especially in a time of heightened immigrant policing, Marta explained. "They think, 'if I call the police on him, my community is going to exclude me.'" This situation is worsened through threats, Marta continued. "Men will say [if you report me], 'I'll tell everyone you put me in jail.'" These threats can be used in conjunction with gendered expectations of women as a form of control, Marta added. "In the rural areas where they're from, your dignity is important. So many women will say, 'I was so afraid because he will say, if I call the police that he's going to tell everybody I was sleeping with another man and that's why he beat me.'" Marta explained that the threat of a damaged reputation is so strong that in some cases this outweighs the concerns about violence. "They would rather deal with the punches than have people think they are sleeping with another man because your dignity is important, and as a woman nobody can think bad about you."

Coercion is a common element in IPV, but immigrant policing can directly shape coercive relationships. For example, abusers may specifically exploit fear related to immigration status and fear of child separation as a form of control, as Lori, a PADV employee, described. "In order to keep them in an abusive situation, abusers will use immigration status against women. They'll say 'they're going to take your children away, and you're going to be back in your country where I know certain people.'" As Lori suggested, some abusers' threats can be transnational. "We had a client who had connections in Mexico, so not only was [the abused partner] being threatened here, but she was also being threatened with her family—her parents in Mexico. So it was like 'yeah, I'll get you deported [here], and over there I can certainly kill you.'"

Marta echoed Lori's comments about how violence extended beyond borders. "Most of the clients, the guys threaten them. [They'll say] 'oh if you go to the police, I'm going to send somebody and hurt your mom or kill your daughter that you left in Mexico.' And believe me, they do." Marta had just finished telling me about a man who had burned down an apartment building with the intention of murdering his girlfriend. Marta's client did not believe her boyfriend would burn down the building, and she was fortunate enough to escape it before it was engulfed in flames. Other threats included targeting parents, siblings, children, and extended family members, and Marta's clients routinely recounted the threats to her: "They'll say 'the next time I called my mom, somebody went to the house and shot the house,' or 'somebody beat my uncle really bad.' So they're thinking 'he means what he says, so I better go back with him.'" These forms of coercion and control could potentially be minimized in the absence of an aggressive immigrant policing regime leading some immigrants to fear reporting violence to police.

In addition to transnational threats and physical violence, some immigrant women also experienced sexual violence and lack of contraceptive choice in their abusive relationships. "I hear it all the time. [They will say,] 'I was having a really hard time with two kids, I don't want another but he would force me.'" Some of Marta's clients ultimately developed strategies for avoiding sex and attempting to control their pregnancies. "I have one client who would say that the way that she would prevent having kids was if the guy didn't come back at Friday at 6:00 pm she knew that he would be drinking. She said every time he would drink he would have sex with her, so she would put five pairs of pants on that night." The goal, for this client, was for her partner to be too drunk to remove five pairs of pants so that he would eventually give up or pass out. This strategy, Marta noted, was necessary because the client was undocumented and could not find contraceptive services, as described in the previous chapter. "That was her pregnancy prevention because she didn't know [what else to do] and she doesn't have access to the services."

As Marta and her clients illustrate, immigration status adds an additional layer of complexity to relationships where some immigrant women must negotiate social networks and violent relationships and find ways to protect themselves. Additionally, immigrant policing directly contributed to risk factors leading to violence, such as economic hardship. As I show in the following section, immigrant policing impacted interpersonal relationships by amplifying factors leading to IPV.

THE ROLE OF IMMIGRANT POLICING IN IPV

Financial stressors are a risk factor for IPV (Capaldi et al. 2012), and as immigrants and service providers noted, immigrant policing directly increased financial stressors in some immigrants' households. As Lori explained, "One of the risk factors [we saw] was if he lost his job or they were going through some sort of health issue or financial problem. The situation here with undocumented immigrants [is that] a lot of people are losing their jobs and being deported, [or they're] not being able to drive to work. It *did* affect domestic violence in the area—we definitely saw it with our clients." Economic tensions were also tied to other risk factors, such as gendered expectations of men in relationships with women. As Lori explained:

"When it comes to domestic violence, [in the 2011 Georgia Domestic Violence Fatality Review Annual Report] they found one of the risk factors came from the idea of affecting gender roles of men, that they need to provide and be strong."

Marta also commented on how immigrant policing regimes contributed to relationship stressors. "I noticed that when the anti-immigrant law passed a lot of people were being laid off. And the violence—the calls we got increased like more than half—the calls, and calls, and calls," Marta said, shaking her head. "I always ask, 'what was he angry about? Why was he angry?' [And the client would say] 'He says it's because he can't find a job; he says it's because he was laid off.' I mean, it's an excuse. It's a valid excuse, but it's an excuse."

The economic challenges resulting from immigrant policing regimes also placed more pressure on some immigrants to not report their abusive partners because they feared loss of income. Some of Marta's clients avoided calling police in a violent situation because they were sure their partners would be deported. "They're very afraid about what's going to happen if he goes to jail and if he's more likely to be deported then who's going to support them? Who's going to feed the kids? And sometimes if they work, the money that they earn is not enough to provide by themselves." Sofia from Caminar Latino also saw examples of men abusing female partners in frustration over lack of work and feeling harassed by police. "Men are angry because they cannot find jobs," she explained, "and the police are harassing them, and they're drinking more because they can't support their families, and then they take it out on their partners." Sofia was quick not to condone abuse, however. "It's not okay, but there are factors that are contributing to this problem," she explained. Immigrant policing exacerbated these concerns among some undocumented couples and families because existing economic instability was made more insecure by intensified policing efforts, such as checkpoints and roadblocks that hindered immigrants' ability to drive without risking detection and deportation.

One of the ways Caminar Latino addressed economic pressures resulting in violence was through group discussions with men who are violent with their partners. "If a man is complaining that he got so angry and frustrated because he hasn't been able to find as much work because he doesn't have papers, and because of the cops being out there, the man right next to him can say, 'I'm experiencing the same thing but you don't see me taking it out on my partner.' . . . They hold each other accountable." To Sofia, the groups provided a way for participants to control how immigrant policing affected their relationships.

Just as economic pressures might make some partners reluctant to call police, some children might also hesitate to call authorities when their parents had fights. As Sofia explained, "One of the things that we found out was that kids were afraid to call the police because they thought that could cause their mom or dad to be deported. The kids were put between a rock and a hard place because they were afraid that their mom was going to either get killed, or that their mom or dad might get deported." Thus immigrant policing affected interpersonal relationships among parents and children in households where violence occurred.

As a result of children hesitating to call police in violent situations, Caminar Latino had to create a violence safety plan that included permission for children to call police if necessary. As part of the new safety plan process, Sofia and her staff met with parents to coach them on how to speak to their children about violence and policing. "We basically meet with the moms beforehand and tell them one of the things that the kids need to hear was that it was okay for them to call the police if they thought their mom was getting hurt or killed because they need to hear it from the parents themselves that it was okay. That they wouldn't get blamed, that they wouldn't get in trouble or anything like that." The revised plans effectively granted children an emotional reprieve from guilt for calling police if violence erupted in their homes.

The threat of deportation was not only a factor that stifled children's willingness to call authorities; it was also a tool of abuse. As Sofia explained, some couples used the threat of deportation as a type of violence. "We see it all the time. He'll threaten to call immigration on her so you'll see he uses her status against her, and she's afraid to call the police because she's afraid of being deported and never seeing her kids again." This type of threat for deportation was especially concerning for mixed-status couples. "If you see that she's undocumented and he's a citizen, there's sometimes a lot of coercion there where he'll threaten to call police on her and have her deported."[4] On the other hand, as Marta explained, women in abusive relationships are sometimes able to use immigrant policing advantageously. Marta will ask her clients if their partners fear police. "And if they say, 'oh yeah, he gets fearful when the police are behind him, he starts shaking,' then I know maybe a restriction order is going to be good for keeping him away.'" Nevertheless, deportation threats as a tool of abuse, children not calling police because they fear parental deportation, and increased economic stressors all point to how immigrant policing efforts aggravate IPV among undocumented immigrants. Similarly, fear of encountering immigration authorities altered some immigrants' willingness to seek IPV services and the way they wanted services provided.

Just as immigrant policing governed immigrants through fear and influenced where some immigrants sought health services, as I described in the previous chapter, it similarly affected how some sought IPV services. As Sofia described, some clients requested new ways of receiving services to reduce their exposure to police: "We see it in terms of people seeking services over the phone now because they're afraid to drive." Marta explained that she ended one of her IPV support groups because participants were too fearful to drive to the meetings. "In 2008, I had a support group, and it was the beginning of when Gwinnett County was applying for the 287(g) [program] . . . A lot of my clients stopped going to the support group until I just had one or two. So I had to stop the groups because nobody was coming." Before ending the support group, Marta called all of the group members to ask whether they would continue coming to the group. "When I called they would say 'you know what, Ms. Marta, I'm afraid to drive over there because my sister-in-law got pulled over and everybody in the car had to show their ID, so I'm not coming anymore because I'm afraid we'll get pulled over.' And so the groups stopped because they were too afraid to drive."

Elaborating on the challenges of getting to group meetings, Lori explained that immigrant policing amplified the negative consequences of having an unreliable mass transportation system, which made it difficult for some of her clients to receive IPV services.

> I had this woman coming to my support group for domestic violence in Gwinnett— poor lady. She was dragging three kids, with a stroller, and the bus there only passed every two hours or so, so she would be late like an hour, and it was either that or be super early an hour, and she would always arrive at the end of my group dragging these children and everything, and she was really tired. She tried so hard because she wanted to be in the support group. She was a nervous wreck, and she really wanted the service. Just by seeing her I would get so exhausted because I know how long the ride was, and carrying three children and everything. That's like a whole day affair just to come to the support group.

Despite being a "whole day affair," taking a bus was the only option for some IPV service seekers since driving was too risky, Lori noted. "People were definitely not taking the risk to drive because they were afraid to get stopped." In one instance, a client was arrested while driving to one of Lori's groups. "This one woman who got stopped while she was driving to us got arrested and her children were there in the car—it was awful."

SYSTEMIC FAILURES IN RESPONDING TO IPV

As already noted, immigrant policing has resulted in heightened distrust between some Latinx communities and law enforcement agencies, making some immigrants more fearful of police and less likely to report crime and victimization. Sofia explained that some police officers recognized how immigrant policing efforts eroded community trust. "One [officer] said, 'we spent so long building a relationship with the Latino community and telling them that they could trust us and telling them that we were here to help, and then this kind of law comes into play and then all of the sudden we're responsible for something we didn't sign up to do. . . .' So now all the work that they did to gain the trust of the Latino community is kind of being thrown out the window." As Lori explained, trust in police is difficult to cultivate among some undocumented Latinx immigrants experiencing IPV because some immigrants who turned to police during violent incidents did not find relief.

Lori recalled an incident with a client who had a violent fight with her husband and feared for her life. "[She] called the police and it was Christmas," Lori explained. "The police came and put [her husband] in the car and they took him around the block, and they talked to him and told him 'you know it's Christmas. Why are you fighting with your wife?' And they turned around and took him back home. And they didn't even make a final report. So she called the police and maybe she's in more danger now, and there's no record of it." While similar situations may occur in relationships with IPV that do not involve immigrants, inappropriately responding to IPV may deepen some immigrants' distrust of law enforcement. Similarly, Sofia claimed some law enforcement agency telephone operators ineffectively responded to immigrants' calls for help by not using the language line translation service when indicated. "Sometimes they call the police and the police don't want to use the language line—a lot of times that happens. So if they call one time and they say they don't speak English, then the police will say 'don't call anymore.'" Police may avoid using the language line because of cost, even though they are provided funds to use the service. This can be even more problematic in relationships where partners have different language abilities, Sofia added, recalling examples of clients who speak only Spanish but whose partners speak English. "A client will say 'I called twice and I can't communicate with the police, and he spoke to them. I don't know what he said, and they didn't do anything, but they let him [back] in the house and he is angrier now.'"

Not taking violence seriously, failing to use available translation services, and inappropriately relying on another person for translation point to ways in which immigration status impacts IPV and how police responses may amplify existing fears about law enforcement agents. Moreover, these situations point to the highly discretionary nature of being a law enforcement agent since officer responses can be inconsistent. Much like the illusory system of health care described in the previous chapter, in some cases, law enforcement agents themselves can become illusory figures, working to purportedly protect all populations but failing to do so. Just as law enforcement officers can fail to protect immigrants, so too can the broader U.S. legal system, as demonstrated by complications in some immigrants getting protection from their abusive situations.

There is a process for undocumented immigrants to be granted relief from their abusers and a legal way to stay in the United States through a U visa. The U visa is a legal authorization reserved for victims of crimes and abuse who aid law enforcement in investigating criminal activity (U.S. Citizenship and Immigration Services, 2018a). The U.S. government sets a cap of granting 10,000 U visas a year; to apply, petitioners must submit relevant credible evidence, a signed statement of victimization, and a certification from a law enforcement official indicating the applicant's assistance with investigating or prosecuting a crime (J. Abrams 2009). After three years of holding a U visa, the visa holder can adjust their status to become a legal permanent resident if they continue to cooperate with law enforcement, but this adjustment is at the discretion of immigration authorities (see U.S. Citizenship and Immigration Services 2018b). The U visa process ultimately uses law enforcement officers as "gatekeepers to the U visa relief" and is problematic because it relies on signing officials' discretion (J. Abrams 2009, 376). This was true for Marta, who explained that some officers were uneasy with signing a document for an immigrant cooperating with investigation of a crime. "Some officers, when they signed the certification, they felt like they were actually the ones giving papers to the person, and they would say 'I don't know this person, they could be a criminal and why would I be signing a document that is basically going to give them papers?'"

As Marta noted, officers were not making immigration determinations; they were instead simply affirming that the petitioner for a U visa reported a crime. But even though U visas are not permanent adjustments to an immigrant's status, some officers refused to sign such affirmations because they did not want to feel responsible for providing an undocumented IPV victim a route to legally stay in the country. This reveals an additional layer of precarity for immigrants in the United States. People who present to police because of IPV or other crimes, like sexual assault, may be subject to disbelief, abuse, and possible homophobic responses (Finneran and Stephenson 2013; Jordan 2004). For immigrants like Marta's client, vulnerability to police disbelief is heightened because it may provide a way for police officers to inquire about immigration status, and in some situations, police officers may not feel inclined to assist an immigrant because of documentation status.

Even with a U visa, the legal system perpetuates vulnerabilities for immigrants seeking relief from IPV. For example, one of Lori's clients came to her seeking protection from an abusive partner who kept her locked in her house with their three children. "One day after he beat her, she escaped and came to our safe house," Lori told me. After getting a U visa, Lori's client went to court to get permanent custody of her children. At the time of her hearing, however, her former partner had recently married a U.S. citizen. "After they had separated, he married an American woman immediately." The relationship ultimately complicated the custody case, Lori explained. "Now it seemed like at least through the eyes of the court, he would be getting his papers soon and she wouldn't." Lori's client had temporary protection with her U visa, and her abusive partner had a route to citizenship through marriage; to the court, marriage seemed a more stable environment for the children. Ultimately immigration authorities came to court and played a role in determining custody. "Long story short," Lori summarized, "her children were taken away from her and she was given a reunification plan in which she was supposed to take English classes, get her GED, go to counseling, get a psych evaluation and get papers. So if she wasn't able to meet those requirements then she wouldn't get her children back." Lori's client felt the burdens were almost insurmountable. "After a while she just felt defeated."

In their work with immigrant women experiencing gender-based partner vio-lence, anthropologists have found that the legal system on which women rely pro-duces a form of structural violence that manifests in few legal options available to those with a precarious immigration status (Parson et al. 2016). There is also limited assistance for navigating the U. S. legal system and understanding its com-plexities (Parson et al. 2016). The situation Lori described further points to how the legal system creates structured inequalities rather than providing reprieve from IPV. It demonstrates how, as critical race scholars have noted (e.g., Bell 1995a, 1995b; Delgado 1995; Freeman 1995), the U.S. legal system can be used to main-tain inequalities rooted in socially driven ideas of difference.

IMMIGRANT POLICING, FEAR, AND INTERPERSONAL RELATIONSHIPS

In this chapter I have described how immigration enforcement regimes directly alter and destabilize interpersonal relationships and can permeate social bound-aries. Focusing on the interpersonal consequences of immigrant policing, and its relationship to IPV, specifically, also reveals failures in the U.S. legal system that could ostensibly provide relief to immigrants who are victims of crimes. As expe-riences like that of Lori's client show, U visas may not always provide a meaning-ful form of relief, as they place immigrants in the system of law enforcement they fear and distrust (Davis 2004), and are available in limited numbers. Few forms of legal relief and an immigration regime that actively works to destabilize rela-tionships point to the emergent need to challenge localized immigrant policing that has long-term impacts on immigrant populations living in the United States.

Through employing fear as a biopolitical technology, immigration enforcement regimes alter undocumented immigrants' individual health behaviors and their interpersonal relationships. Moreover, as I show in the next chapter, immigrant policing also affects health providers' professional practices. However, just as undocumented immigrants resisted the interpersonal consequences of immigrant policing through teatros and similar actions, providers also found ways to com-bat immigration enforcement regimes and resist forms of professional control.

5 · "A DEATH BY A THOUSAND LITTLE CUTS"

Health Providers and Immigrant Policing

When I walked into the Healing Grace of God (HGG) clinic, I was struck by the size and newness of the facility.[1] I had visited clinics run by faith-based organizations during fieldwork in Florida on different projects related to immigrant and farmworker health, but none of the facilities I had seen were nearly as nice or new as this Atlanta clinic. As I waited at the front desk to speak to someone behind a sliding-glass window, I peered around the bright, well-lit room. GLAHRiadores and members of the Hispanic Health Coalition of Georgia (HHCGA), a nonprofit organization that held annual health fairs, screenings, and health promotion events, had suggested that I reach out to HGG, claiming it was a place numerous undocumented Latinx immigrants went for care. After checking in at the front desk, I looked for a seat in the half-full waiting room—the size of a university classroom that could accommodate fifty students. Nearly every vacant seat had a Bible on it. As I sat down, I scanned the walls, which were adorned with crosses and images of angels. After a few minutes, a nurse summoned me to Dr. Taylor's private office.

I sat at a conference table near the door, waiting for Dr. Taylor, counting the numerous running medals, triathlon awards, race photos, and framed marathon participant stickers hanging on the drywall. Several minutes later, Dr. Taylor, founder of HGG, entered the room carrying a plate with his lunch. "Sorry to keep you waiting. So you're wanting to talk about illegal immigrants and health care?" Dr. Taylor took a seat and almost immediately cut into his food. I explained my project and asked about HGG, which had opened in the mid-1990s as a place where low-income individuals could receive preventive medical care, prenatal care, counseling, and dental services. As our conversation turned to undocumented immigrants and Georgia's well-known anti-immigrant law, HB 87, Dr. Taylor shared some of his frustrations with immigrant policing.

"We have a ton of illegal patients but we don't identify them, and I'll tell you why we don't. It has nothing to do with a view of public policy—it has *nothing* to do with that. My view is that first of all it's the government's job to police the borders; it is not my job. That's why I pay taxes. . . . *It's not my job to police the borders!*" After elaborating on how he viewed the current immigration situation as a result of federal inaction, corporations wanting cheap labor, and individual immigrants wanting to improve their economic circumstances, Dr. Taylor explained that he would provide care for patients regardless of their immigration status. "Our job is once the person is here and they want health care, to provide it. For example," Dr. Taylor continued fervently, "a mother with a little baby who's six months old and has a 103-degree fever appears at my doorstep. Well that little child doesn't have any control over his situation. He didn't ask to be where he is right now; he didn't ask to be sick!"

Using the febrile child as an example, Dr. Taylor continued to explain why he felt it was important to provide care to any patient regardless of immigration status. "We feel like it's our moral obligation to do what we can to try to take care of that child within our scope and ability." Beyond simply caring for a child who "didn't choose to be sick," Dr. Taylor further explained his motivations as a physician being rooted in his faith.

> We feel like we should be doing this because of the idea of service. Most of these people, directly or indirectly, are serving me, so we're serving them back. And you could say that's biblical, well it is biblical, moral and biblical. Those are people who are cleaning my yard; they're blowing leaves off my yard, or they put a roof on the house of the people who lost it because of the tornadoes last week, or they're picking the vegetables that appear at my grocery store. So this is our way of serving them and again it goes back to that moral of that person who appears at our doorstep and is sick and needs help. So we feel like *that's* our job—not policing the border.

Throughout our interview, Dr. Taylor attempted to anticipate my questions and reiterated his disinterest in determining patients' immigration status. "Now you are probably going to ask the question 'do we document people' [ask for their immigration status], and no, we don't. Again, because it's my philosophy that it's not my job, it's the government's job to police the borders, *it is not my job*!! So I'm not going to do that." Dr. Taylor then clarified that he assesses his employees' immigration status, but not his patients'. "We hire people who are here and legally able to work in this country, but as far as who we treat, they choose to come here and if they need us and their baby needs care, we take care of them."

As described in chapter 2, federal and state statutes require all employers, including HGG, to assess a potential employee's immigration status, and HB 87 had initially made it a crime for providers to use public funds to treat undocumented patients until an intermediate appellate court overturned that specific portion of the law. Expressing his concerns with how immigrant policing and laws like HB 87 impacted providers and his organization, Dr. Taylor argued that assessing a patient's immigration status was an inappropriate use of his time.

> This stuff about not treating people because they're illegal—the thing about being a physician or dentist or whoever, is that our education and skill set is really to take care of a person. If we all of the sudden have to start trying to assess whether someone's here legally or not, you're robbing me of doing what I do well and therefore you're robbing time from me, and therefore that's a patient I can't see because I'm taking the time to do something else! If you think about time, resources, and skill sets, and things like that, it's a bad use of skill sets for me to be doing that. And then you can say "okay well you can ask your staff to do that." Well if I'm asking my staff to do that, again I'm asking somebody to give their time, if everybody who comes through that door is being checked, we have to hire a whole other person to do that. You have to hire that whole other person and I have to pay that person, and again that's money that I can use for some other purpose, such as hiring another doctor. So again, that would be fewer patients that I would be able to see.

Dr. Taylor's assertions of how immigrant policing and HB 87, specifically, impinged on his professional practice mirror other providers' feelings. Several providers I met in Atlanta expressed a sense of outrage or inappropriateness with legislation interfering with their professional practice and prohibiting them from providing certain types of care to undocumented patients. Additionally, some providers commented on how immigrant policing regimes affected their entire practices, as Dr. Taylor alluded to when he discussed the inefficiencies of using providers to assess patients' immigration statuses. Although Dr. Taylor's motivations for treating undocumented immigrants were partly informed by a religious perspective not shared by other providers, his sense of outrage that legislators would impose on his professional practice was a common theme.

In this chapter, I show how immigrant policing directly affected health providers and describe how some providers resisted policing efforts. I also discuss how immigration enforcement efforts ultimately result in what one provider called "a death by a thousand little cuts": subtle ways of creating harm that aggregate to larger consequences. The metaphorical "death by a thousand cuts" alludes to how immigrant policing efforts operate on numerous fronts, impacting immigrants' individual health behaviors and mobility, interpersonal relationships, and the providers with whom they may come into contact. I further show how immigrant policing efforts operate in ways that push some providers into complying with neoliberal frameworks for providing health care, revealing how immigrant policing efforts guide not only some immigrants' conduct, as I described in chapter 3, but providers' as well.

IMMIGRANT POLICING AND HEALTH PROVIDERS

As already described, the immigrant policing regime in Georgia comprises state and federal laws and police officers' actions, like setting up checkpoints and requesting proof of legal status from someone suspected of being undocumented. The most well-known state law, HB 87, contributed to the complex web of immigration enforcement in Georgia but also affected health providers in two ways. First, the law restricted health care workers' ability to provide certain types of care to undocumented immigrants, and second, HB 87 created new requirements for providers to renew their professional licenses (see chapter 2). These two factors resulted in health providers being implicated in and feeling the consequences of immigrant policing.

As I described in chapter 1, when HB 87 passed, it specifically expanded definitions of "harboring an illegal alien" to include "any conduct that tends to substantially help an illegal alien to remain in the United States," such as using public funds to provide nonemergency health services to undocumented immigrants. This provision potentially meant providers on a public entity's payroll, like a state health department or public hospital, could be arrested for providing care to an undocumented immigrant. The law could also be interpreted to include private facilities that receive public funds in the form of grants or see documented patients who pay for services using public funds like Medicaid or Medicare. Overall, then, the breadth of the provisions possibly implicated the majority of providers in Georgia. Although an intermediate appellate court struck the provision related to health providers, it nevertheless had legislators' support and passed with the language restricting providers' ability to care for undocumented immigrants in nonemergency situations.

In addition to criminalizing certain types of care, HB 87 created new hurdles for providers renewing their professional licenses (see chapter 2). In Georgia, physicians and nurses, specifically, must renew their professional licenses every two years. HB 87 required that all professionals, regardless of immigration or citizenship status, submit proof of legal status to the Georgia secretary of state when renewing their professional license. To complete their license renewal, citizens and noncitizens alike were required to submit a copy of a U.S.-government-issued photo identification, and noncitizens were further required to submit documents from federal immigration authorities. The requirements resulted in large delays in license renewals and overwhelmed the secretary of state's office, which has the responsibility of verifying licensees' legal status.

The inability of the secretary of state to keep up with license renewal demands resulted in the Georgia Composite Medical Board, the state agency that grants professional licenses to physicians, reporting that at one point in time, at least 1,300 medical professionals lost their legal ability to practice (Burress 2012).[2] Further, the secretary of state, which oversees licenses for nurses, placed holds on 3,500 nurses because they were unable to verify their legal status (Crawford 2013)—a considerable problem since the state faces a shortage of nurses (A. Miller 2017). The administrative hurdles in renewing licenses remained a concern for providers until 2013, when SB 160, as described in chapter 2, went into effect, and required a onetime legal status verification to be sufficient instead of verification with every renewal. Nevertheless, the licensure changes associated with HB 87 created widespread administrative concerns at hospitals and among providers.

One provider, Dr. Bazil, recalled the disturbance the licensing requirement changes created at the hospital where he worked. Commenting on his hospital's response to the licensing problem, he noted the institution's internal panic: "We got this email from HR and they were freaking out about us needing to renew our licenses immediately." The urgency struck Dr. Bazil as odd. "Usually you just do it one or two weeks before it expires, but I guess that wasn't working anymore because there were people who submitted the renewal and it didn't go through in time." The lack of a prompt license renewal meant that providers in Dr. Bazil's hospital legally lost their ability to work because of the delays that HB 87 caused. "So they literally were working their shift and their license expired and they had to stop. So after that, everyone freaked out and they started making us renew our license months ahead of time."

Another provider, Dr. Manheim, who worked at Grady Memorial Hospital, was unsure why new procedures were in place when he had to renew his license. "I got this email not too long ago where they were asking me for a copy of my passport. I've never had to do it before, and I remember thinking that was odd. I thought it was strange at the time, but it sort of makes sense now that I think about it with this law." Dr. Manheim is an immigrant who moved to the United States with his family when he was a child. When he received the email about having to show his passport he initially assumed it was because of his ethnicity. "When I first got it I thought 'is it because I'm Arab? Would they ask my [non-Arab] boss to show a passport?'" Dr. Manheim continued to explain that changes in licensing requirements do not necessarily harm individual providers but instead affect the entire institution, particularly a large hospital like his. "For each provider individually it's certainly not a big deal if you make a photocopy of your passport and turn it in. On an institutional level though, and at a hospital like this one, in particular, with so many doctors, it can create a lot of turmoil." Dr. Manheim recalled hearing about licensing changes when HB 87 was discussed in the media, but did not pay much attention to the specifics. He, like many other providers, considered HB 87 an unnecessary, if not upsetting, measure of oversight that impinged on providers' professional duties. "A lot of this stuff is stupid," he said, "so what's the point?"

Medical professionals are subjected to numerous types of oversight and control designed to protect patients, providers, and health organizations and corporations from various types of harm. HB 87 added a layer of control over medical professionals that providers I interviewed actively resisted. Complicating providers' practice by creating immigration-related licensure hurdles and criminalizing the kind of care they can provide to immigrant patients represent efforts to incorporate immigration enforcement objectives into medical regulatory regimes. As I show in this chapter, immigrant policing has numerous impacts on providers, and like immigrants, providers can resist immigration enforcement efforts.

WITCH HUNTS AND INCREDULITY

Although health providers in the United States are accustomed to regulatory regimes and biomedical bureaucracies like licensures, diagnostic codes, health insurance requirements, and statutes governing professional expectations, several health care professionals were disturbed by the way HB 87 added immigration matters to providers' sphere of regulatory concerns. Providers were incensed by the original language of HB 87, which could result in medical providers being charged with a crime for treating undocumented patients. Health professionals I spoke with in Atlanta felt HB 87 would have been unenforceable and was an encroachment on professional responsibilities, echoing Dr. Taylor's comments. One physician, Dr. West, expressed outrage and incredulity about the legislature interfering with providers' work in ways that HB 87 did. "That somebody would have the balls to put that in legislation—that's disturbing," Dr. West said. Despite an appellate court throwing out the provision of HB 87 that directly constrained health workers' legal ability to provide certain types of care, Dr. Manheim, like Dr. West, was alarmed by such extreme measures to regulate providers. "Ultimately it obviously got thrown out [the provision about providing care], so I think that was certainly the right thing to do, but the fact that even sort of made it [into the law in the first place] is kind of ridiculous and terrifying."

In addition to being incredulous about HB 87 and its impact on health professionals, Dr. Manheim found HB 87 impossible to enforce. "Honestly," Dr. Manheim explained, "I think it would be one of those things that if they did actually prosecute someone for, first of all who would do that, and second of all, what would happen from a community perspective to say to people 'this is really what happened: a doctor was arrested for taking care of a patient?' Well, that's their job." Another provider at a large Atlanta-area hospital, Dr. Pfeiffer, explained that he would not refuse care to any patients, and that a legislative attempt to require him to do so was inappropriate. "I have to report potential harm or danger to self or others. It's not appropriate to report immigration status. . . . [lack of] Citizenship is not a duty to warn [issue]." As Dr. Pfeiffer alluded to, health care providers may have a professional and ethical "duty to warn" third parties about potential harms a patient may cause themselves or others.[3] Providers must also report certain infectious diseases, such as tuberculosis and HIV, to state authorities, but immigration status is not a serious harm and there is no "duty to warn" expectation around immigration matters.

Beyond viewing provisions in HB 87 as unenforceable or encroaching on professional responsibilities, some providers I spoke to had responses informed by notions of humanitarianism, similar to Dr. Taylor's, but not guided by religious beliefs. One provider at a teaching hospital, for example, said, "I see a patient, students see a patient—I don't care what their immigration status is, they are *human beings*. They have something that we can take care of and that is our job. It is not to judge; it is not to inquire." For this provider, all human beings deserved care, regardless of citizenship status.

In explaining the focus of laws like HB 87, some providers felt that the law was a "witch hunt" driven by racist attitudes. As one physician, Dr. Layne, who moved to Atlanta in 2006, explained, "I think it's this knee-jerk conservatism, well, racism. I'll call a spade a spade, I think that's what it is—it's not economic; that's their very transparent coverup. Laws like these are racist." Dr. Layne continued to explain that she saw historical similarities between how immigrants in Georgia were targeted by laws like HB 87 and how other minority groups systematically lost their rights. "If you look at our history there have been some situations where this is how it starts, you know? It's a witch hunt: people who look like this or are this religion or this orientation, you can't help them. And then it becomes you can't just help them, you have to *get* them. And that's my fear: that we're moving from 'just don't harbor them in your home or help them' to '*get them!*'"

Echoing Dr. Layne, a nurse at one of Georgia's health departments, Jane, expressed a similar but bleaker perspective. "To me it just harkens [to] pre-Nazi Germany. People are hurting, we have a bad economy, things aren't going right for people, and it's really easy to galvanize around some group [or] other. Right now our 'other' is people south of the American border." Moreover, Jane commented on how such efforts can distract from other political problems, such as failing economic policy. "Don't worry about how we are screwing you over in all of these other ways, don't look at that, look at the shiny thing over here. Blame these people for taking that tomato-picking job that I'm sure you weren't going to take because I don't know any Americans that pick produce other than high school kids picking watermelon in Florida in the summer."

Dr. West felt the nature of the medical profession potentially limited providers' involvement in political processes, which, in his opinion, explained laws like HB 87. "The problem with physicians," he explained, "and I think it's a generalization, but I think it's why we are where we are in health care, is that we are so busy and overwhelmed with the care of medicine that politics and these other things . . . we don't have time for it." A lack of time was largely because of the immediate needs of patients, Dr. West argued. "You know, we've got patients to see and that's really killed us because we don't stand up and fight for things, and it's not because we don't care, it's because we've got another patient in front of us.

And I think that's a sad reality and that's why we're pushed around by some of these crazy ass policies coming out of DC and our [state] administration. We essentially have no voice on the Hill [i.e., U.S. Congress]."

Although Dr. West argued that providers had little political influence on immigration issues, there are examples of health-related professional organizations acting on immigration. For instance, the American Academy of Pediatrics issued a statement in 2017 asserting the organization's view that immigration policies from the Trump administration were harmful to children's health (Stein 2017). Similarly, in 2018, the American Medical Association released a letter urging the Trump administration to end the zero tolerance policy resulting in family separation, as described in the previous chapter (Madara 2018). These examples represent small efforts from professional groups that individual providers could continue to promote in local settings. In Georgia, some students training to become health professionals actively fought for political causes through Health Students Taking Action Together (HealthSTAT).

HealthSTAT lobbies for or against specific pieces of health-related legislation. The organization is composed of medical, nursing, physical therapy, pharmacy, public health, law, and business students from Emory University, Georgia State University, Medical College of Georgia, Mercer University, Morehouse School of Medicine, and Philadelphia College of Osteopathic Medicine (which operates a campus in an Atlanta suburb). As part of its routine lobbying efforts, HealthSTAT conducts advocacy training and organizes breakfasts with Georgia legislators for its members. When I met leaders of HealthSTAT in January 2013, the organization's main focus was to encourage policy makers to expand Medicaid, reflecting a national debate about the Patient Protection and Affordable Care Act, the United States' most recent health reform law.

Every legislative season, HealthSTAT leaders chose different issues on which to focus, such as gun violence prevention, exercise promotion, and increasing the tobacco tax. When we met, immigration was not a key priority, but in 2005 and 2006, HealthSTAT had focused on immigrant health and vocally opposed anti-immigrant legislation, taking direct action against one of Georgia's early anti-immigrant laws, SB 529. Early versions of this law would have required verification of legal status before a person received publicly funded health services, and HealthSTAT leaders argued the law placed an unnecessary burden on health care workers. In response, they organized 150 medical students from across the state to attend a rally on the steps of the capitol, donning their white lab coats, and demanding that health care be exempted from SB 529 (Health Students Taking Action Together 2016). "The day we got everyone to wear their white coats and show up to the capitol," one HealthSTAT leader, finishing his medical education, recalled, "that was amazing. We were all there and you couldn't miss us because of our coats." Ultimately SB 529 passed with prenatal care, pediatric care, and emergency services being excepted from the requirement to verify legal status before receiving care (Health Students Taking Action Together 2016).

The HealthSTAT example demonstrates how students in health-related programs were able to resist efforts to use health professionals as a tool for immigrant policing. Additionally, providers in Atlanta discussed how they actively resisted immigration enforcement regimes encroaching on their occupation. Forms of resistance demonstrated how some providers could reject participation in what they saw as "witch hunts" or refuse to be complicit with laws they found suspicious. In some situations, however, health professionals were unsure of how immigration enforcement laws impacted them, prompting local groups like the HHCGA to engage in awareness efforts.

ER DOUBLE CHECKS, A WILLINGNESS TO BE ARRESTED, AND "DON'T ASK, DON'T TELL"

In Atlanta, some providers rejected the notion that immigrant policing efforts should limit their professional roles, and in some cases, this included defiantly interpreting elements of HB 87. For example, providers such as Dr. Taylor interpreted HB 87's requirements for not using public funds to treat undocumented immigrants as restricting the government from writing a check for a service. As Dr. Taylor said, "If the government's paying for it they can say it's illegal, but they're not paying for it. So if you've provided nonemergency services for someone and the government's not paying for it, and the patient *is* paying for it, we have not violated the law." In other words, to Dr. Taylor, criminalizing efforts to provide publicly funded services to immigrants was moot since immigrants paid for their services, regardless of how a facility received funding.

Further pointing to what he viewed as the absurd exclusion of emergency care, Dr. Taylor noted that many people used the emergency room as a source of primary care because they lacked health insurance or lacked other ways of seeing a provider and financing health services in the United States' market-based medical system. "It depends on how you define an emergency because a lot of people use the *emergency room*," Dr. Taylor said in an exaggerated way, using air quotes, "for their primary care, when in reality what they're having is not a real 'emergency.' But they still use the emergency room for their primary care, so what's the emergency room supposed to do about that? Sometimes they have a hard time turning people away—they're there, and they're sick." As Dr. Taylor suggested, all emergency room physicians I spoke with mentioned they would not turn away patients even if they were not experiencing a medical emergency.

Commenting on emergency room providers generally, one ER physician, Dr. Drake, explained that he had no interest in determining a patient's citizenship before providing care. "Particularly in the emergency department, and it probably gets us in trouble, but we tend to be pretty altruistic. We tend not to worry about somebody's citizenship. In general, we're going to take care of everybody regardless of race, creed, color, whatever the case may be. So things like the bill, and immigration, and checkpoints, we tend not to think about that at all, quite honestly." Dr. Drake explained that although citizenship or legal status considerations do not impact how he provides care, they will influence how he recommends follow-up care. "When we have to think about the follow-up plan, we do have to think about [legal status and ability to pay] a little bit at least because we have to understand what a patient can and cannot afford, we have to think about where we can send them, and those kinds of things. . . . Rarely do we ask about citizenship per se."

While providing emergency care was not criminalized by HB 87, Dr. Drake noted he would provide care through the emergency room regardless of any immigration law, even if the laws eventually did include emergent care. "They're not going to stop me from treating a patient that comes into our ER, regardless of citizenship, ability to pay, whatever." This type of assertion suggested how providers like Dr. Drake and others can resist efforts to encroach on their professional actions. One of the most salient examples of how this type of resistance can work is the ways in which some physicians at Grady Memorial Hospital double-checked the symptoms of undocumented patients of chronic kidney failure when they reported to the emergency room.

In 2009, Grady closed its outpatient dialysis center, jeopardizing the lives of fifty-one kidney failure patients, nearly all undocumented (Kline 2018c; Rodriguez 2015; Sack 2009b).[4] Kidney failure is fatal and requires dialysis two or three times a week or a kidney transplant to survive (Centers for Disease Control and Prevention 2014; LaRocco 2011). Dialysis is more common than transplantation, and the process involves removing blood from the body, passing it through a filtering machine, and pumping it back into the body to keep a patient alive. When Grady closed its dialysis facility, it placed some patients in private, for-profit dialysis centers and medically repatriated others to their countries of birth (Sack 2009a). Some undocumented kidney failure patients, however, reported to Grady's emergency department for care because they had nowhere else to go, and without treatment, they would die on average within ten days (*New York Times* 2009).

Uninsured indigent patients who report to hospitals with life-threatening conditions are able to receive a limited form of publicly funded health services through a special type of Medicaid program called Emergency Medicaid. The program reimburses hospitals for treating patients who present with an emergent condition: a health issue with a "sudden onset" that may result in serious dysfunction or death (Rodriguez 2010), such as shortness of breath or symptoms of a heart attack. Through Emergency Medicaid, uninsured U.S. residents can get care in urgent situations, which, as anthropologist Heide Castañeda has noted, permits, "massive opposition to universal health care, while still allowing Americans to 'sleep easy' because no one is dying in the streets" (2010, 13). However, some illnesses, like kidney failure, are life-threatening but are not necessarily considered "emergent conditions" because they are chronic (Rodriguez 2010), and therefore they are not regarded as Emergency Medicaid exceptions. Excluding diseases that are swiftly fatal but chronic from definitions of emergent results in a heightened vulnerability to death among indigent and uninsured patients, like undocumented immigrants.

After Grady closed its outpatient dialysis center and placed patients in different facilities, ten to twelve undocumented patients continued seeking care through the Grady ER. Because of how "emergent" is defined, undocumented patients could not receive dialysis without having a medical emergency that first required hospital admission. As a medical social worker at Grady, Aricél, noted, "If it's not an emergency then we are supposed to discharge them. So if they don't have an indication for anything emergent we can't admit them for routine dialysis." If patients lack an emergent condition, staff and providers must suggest patients return when they are closer to death. As Aricél explained: "So we do from time to time send [the undocumented patients] back home and we tell them basically, I mean, I hate it, but we tell them 'when you're sicker, come back' because they don't have access to services."

As Aricél explained to me, statutory definitions of "emergent" have created requirements where undocumented patients must be as close to death as possible in order to receive dialysis. Receiving treatment therefore involves a costly and inefficient process in which patients are sometimes pushed to the brink of death so that they can be admitted to the hospital for a condition considered emergent, then they can be stabilized, and then they are able to receive dialysis as part of their stabilization. The process then restarts as soon as a patient is discharged from the hospital. As a Grady provider summarized the situation, "All these patients have to be admitted to the hospital, so they get admitted in the ER and are usually here for a day or two. Then they go home, and then they come back a couple of days later, so unfortunately it's this never-ending vicious circle."

The vicious cycle the provider described places undocumented immigrants in a liminal state between life and death, needing constant intervention to survive. Such liminal forms of life, as philosopher Achille Mbembe argues, are a result of political subjugation that blurs the boundaries between life and death, a type of "necropolitics" or "death-in-life" (Mbembe and Meintjes 2003, 21). In the case of undocumented kidney failure patients, they are left in a position of what medical anthropologist Miriam Ticktin has called "the living dead": "a state that, in the immediacy and intensity of their struggle for survival, is indistinguishable from the threat of physical death" (2006, 42).

If the patient does not have an emergent condition, the hospital cannot provide emergency care and be reimbursed for the costs. This problem ultimately led some emergency room providers to double-check with patients before sending them home and telling them to "come back when [they are] sicker." Some providers made absolutely sure patients did not experience symptoms of an emergent condition before discharging them, since without these conditions patients must wait until they are ill enough to warrant receiving emergency treatment. As one provider, Dr. Mason, explained, "[To be sure they are not experiencing an emergency] we'll say, 'are you having shortness of breath? Are you having chest pains?' but if not, we have to send them home." Running through such a checklist allows providers to be certain their patients are not turned away without exhausting an option to treat them.

The Grady dialysis situation demonstrates the arbitrary nature of defining diseases based on chronicity, and underscores, as anthropologists Lenore Manderson and Carolyn Smith-Morris have argued, that "increasingly, chronic, long-term conditions are not naturally occurring ones, but are those for which the political will and economic resources are simply not brought to bear for a given community" (2010, 18). Some individual providers can resist political constraints on providing care to kidney failure patients by taking extra measures to be certain patients are not inadvertently excluded from a possible source of care. Other providers echoed this point and were even willing to be arrested for providing the type of care they thought was necessary to their patients.

In addition to finding ways to resist immigrant policing efforts, some providers expressed positions of defiance to immigrant policing. In expressing her personal refusal to comply with laws like HB 87, Dr. Hernandez, whom I described in the previous chapter, said, "I don't really pay any attention to whether it's a law now or not a law. I'm going to give care no matter what. If I could get fined or arrested because of that, that's just how it's going to be, but I think I speak for a lot of my colleagues, too." Another provider, Dr. Smith, explained legislation would not change who he treated, and if anything, he and other providers would view such legislation as a challenge. "It wouldn't affect what I did. It might criminalize what I *do*, but there's a higher purpose, so I'd be happy to be taken to court. Let somebody try to throw me in jail for doing the right thing. I think in that sense it was almost a challenge. There was never a sense of panic over it," Dr. Smith explained.

Like Dr. Smith and Dr. Hernandez, Dr. Tobias refused to comply with HB 87 even if the provisions criminalizing care to undocumented immigrants remained in the law. Having lived in Atlanta for nearly thirty years and considering himself politically engaged, Dr. Tobias noted that no piece of legislation would prevent him from seeing undocumented patients. His rationale was partly because he felt laws like HB 87 were written by Republican legislators who represented the interests of conservative suburban residents, and not the interests of everyone in the Atlanta area. "These suburbs are just incredibly different from anything I was ever raised in. It's this 'I got stuff, I don't want you to have it, and I'm afraid you're going to get it' mentality. 'I struggled to get what I got,' and all that kind of stuff. 'We have traditions here,' and that kind of thing. People who like things the way they are don't want them to change." As I explained in chapter 1, Atlanta's immigrant population largely settled in suburban areas; and as I described in chapter 2, political leaders from these areas helped draft some of Georgia's immigrant policing statutes, including HB 87. Reiterating points from providers such as Dr. Layne, who viewed laws like HB 87 through a racial lens, Dr. Tobias explained the legislation in terms of Georgia's suburban expansion linked to its history of racial tension, explaining that suburban politicians used immigration laws to appeal to white voters concerned over the growing Latino population in Atlanta. "Stuff like this is just class warfare and racism. . . . That's always the subtext; it's always racial, but those people are probably clever enough not to make it obvious."

Dr. Tobias noted that the racial implications of laws like HB 87 dismiss the economic contribution immigrants have made to Atlanta. "The economic boost immigrants provide is incalculable. They've built every structure in Atlanta in the last 50 years. Those buildings would not be there if it wasn't for that cheap labor, and how can you not understand that? That's the part that I don't get. That's who mows your yard, for God's sake!" Because of what he viewed as policies intended to protect interests of suburban, affluent, white residents, Dr. Tobias explained that he paid no attention to laws like HB 87 that limited his professional practice because of what he viewed as racist sentiments. "I see plenty of people who are undocumented, for sure. . . . I think people in Atlanta realize those guys [legislators who co-wrote HB 87] from the suburbs are nuts." For Dr. Tobias, then, HB 87 lacked legitimacy in part because it represented racist interests from leaders he did not identify with, in addition to violating professional obligations to treat patients.

Medical anthropologists have described how providers' professional activities can be managed by a power regime that promotes a specific agenda, and how providers can directly object to impositions on their professional practice (see, for example, Mishtal 2009). In Atlanta, some providers, such as Dr. Hernandez and Dr. Smith, have expressed direct objections to immigrant policing efforts imposing on their professional practice. Furthermore, providers such as Dr. Taylor and others specifically argued how efforts to criminalize some of their professional behaviors were unacceptable and interfered with personal and professional ethics. Dr. Taylor even noted how such efforts were counterproductive to his practice. Moreover, providers such as Dr. Tobias questioned the legitimacy of laws driven by racism. These rationales all demonstrate how providers can resist immigrant policing efforts by using their own professional positions of authority. Health providers are granted a great deal of social and cultural authority based on their capacities to define life, death, and disease in institutions that provide systems of rules and organization, such as hospitals (Posner, Gild, and Winans 1995). When exposed to new types of bureaucratic order, providers can assert or maintain their authority by using medical knowledge and professional judgment related to care (Posner, Gild, and Winans 1995). In Atlanta, health care providers assert both humanitarian and professional judgment arguments against immigrant policing efforts, and providers can continue to resist immigration enforcement efforts at state and federal levels, as I argue in chapter 7.

Although some providers expressed resistance and opposition to provisions in HB 87 that would restrict to whom they offered care, other providers explained that there was a sense of confusion among providers. One community health advocate, Marco, who works for a large, private hospital, explained that many providers and community health workers at his hospital are unsure about whether providing care or organizing health promotion events is legal. "There's still a big 'don't ask, don't tell' part of it," he said, referencing a former U.S. military policy regarding service members' sexual orientation. "People are a lot more guarded. The providers have this idea that they know they're doing the right thing because they're treating somebody that needs it, but they wonder if they can get in trouble for it." Potential repercussions for providing treatment weighed on some staff, and some hospital officials had concerns over whether they were permitted to treat patients, as Marco said. "Nobody knows what's legal and what's not. We don't know if we're doing something we can get arrested for or not." Providers' uncertainty about the legality of providing care to undocumented patients resulted in the HHCGA finding information regarding immigration laws, interpreting how they impacted providers, and distributing the information to members.

The HHCGA comprised health providers, staff from Atlanta's major hospitals, academic researchers, public health students and practitioners, and individuals interested in promoting Latinx health needs. Members worked to share information and to design programs focused on four key themes the coalition identified as areas of need: cardiovascular health, diabetes, and obesity; cancer; maternal and child health; and behavioral health. Members of the coalition met in task forces focused on these topics to discuss possible interventions and ways to address identified problems. During my fieldwork, I attended HHCGA events and quarterly meetings and was an active member of the task forces on cancer and maternal and child health because of my experience working on those topics as a public health graduate student.

Because the task force members and organization leaders were aware of my fieldwork, I was asked to work on the HHCGA's immigration law project with a graduate student pursuing a public health degree at Emory University. The result of our collaboration was a list of immigration laws and their impact on immigrants and providers, as well as the long-term consequences of these laws on both providers and immigrants. With this list, the HHCGA cancer committee developed potential action plans to disseminate information to *promotoras* (lay community health workers), providers, and organizations that provide cancer screening services or provide low-cost or subsidized care in an effort to assuage potential fears about seeking and providing care.[5] Although the fact sheet for the HHCGA is an example of how some organizations can combat how immigrant policing affects providers, it nevertheless is not a full answer to the broader problem of destabilizing immigrants' communities and institutions they may seek assistance from.

"DEATH BY A THOUSAND LITTLE CUTS" AND CONSEQUENCES FOR CLINICAL PRACTICE

In reflecting on how immigrant policing affected providers and immigrants alike, one provider noted how immigration enforcement efforts were ways of slowly eroding immigrants' stability in the United States. Dr. Green, a provider who has lived in Atlanta since the 1990s, argued that immigration enforcement laws represented smaller, rationalized ways of reducing health care to certain populations. These types of laws made the results of decreasing services and concomitant worsened health outcomes more acceptable among the public. "There's no watershed moment," he argued. "So you don't go from offering something to not offering *anything*. There's very rarely a dramatic moment like that where you can say 'that death was due to this [denying undocumented immigrants care].' It's a death by a thousand little cuts. It's hard to really document or show the effect of something like this." For Dr. Green, the consequence of immigrant policing, a "death by a thousand little cuts," fits squarely within the aims of interior immigration enforcement efforts that attempt to make life so challenging for immigrants that they choose to "self-deport." From Dr. Green's explanation, restrictions in types of care that could be provided was one of the thousand or more cuts that may encourage "self-deportation."

Gradually stripping away services available for undocumented immigrants allows for a slow, acceptable process of denying sets of rights and entitlements, or broadly denying immigrants' "medical citizenship" (Horton 2014): a sense of belonging to formal medical institutions. A "death by a thousand cuts" demonstrates the gradual processes of formally denying medical citizenship to undocumented immigrants and further speaks to how laws like HB 87 may advance efforts to promote immigrant attrition, suggesting how medical professions can be used as part of legislators' attrition goal. Criminalizing types of care available to undocumented immigrants is one of the "thousand cuts" to promote immigrant attrition, but it also serves to deny undocumented immigrants' health-related rights, thus creating ways to formally deny potential claims to medical citizenship.

While a "death by a thousand cuts" directly impacted undocumented immigrants, immigration enforcement regimes that create such cuts also impacted providers' clinical operations. Some health professionals I met in Atlanta explained that the consequences of immigrant policing led them to change how they offered services. In one example, immigrant policing directly changed practices in a clinical setting. Dr. Arias, a mental health provider at the Center for Education, Treatment, and Prevention of Addiction (CETPA), explained that immigrant policing regimes impacted his practice. "The number one reason for people not showing up for their appointments here," he said, as we sat in his office, "is that they're afraid to drive because they're afraid they're going to be pulled over." Intense fear of being pulled over that resulted in not showing up for appointments was a new problem for his clients, he explained. "Before all these immigration laws, we had a very low no-show rate." Another counselor at CETPA added to this, explaining that no-show rates increase during times when police are more active. "During the summertime there are just a lot more cops out there checking for speeding and when people realize what's going on, one person tells another there's a cop on [Interstate] 85, or there's a cop outside and people stay home. We have this no-show rate that's extremely high during the summertime," the counselor said. "When we ask 'why,' they will tell us 'well you know cops are everywhere, so we can't leave the house; we're going to get pulled over.'"

Continuing to explain how patients were affected by immigration laws, Dr. Arias noted that all family members, regardless of documentation status, felt the impacts of immigrant policing. "We hear the stories that police have parked cars outside of the church, or the police have parked cars outside of school, so people don't want to drive. . . . So a couple of things we discovered: not only is the undocumented person unable to now go seek services, but we're finding that they're living in a mixed household with mixed levels of documentation status, and the ones that have documentation will also avoid going to the doctor." Avoidance, as Dr. Arias noted, was partly to protect family members. "The reason we're seeing this is that people don't want to do anything that will draw attention to themselves and get a question about who lives with you, and they don't put their family members in jeopardy."

Medical anthropologists and other social scientists have shown how immigration policies impact families that have numerous status configurations. A single household can feature a constellation of immigration statuses, and any type of status vulnerability can impact the entire family (Castañeda 2019; Vargas and Pirog 2016; Castañeda and Melo 2014). As Dr. Arias indicated, in some circumstances, documented household members might avoid seeking services in order to protect members of the entire household (Miklavcic 2011). Accordingly, as I noted in the previous chapter, immigrant policing efforts can disrupt numerous interpersonal relationships, but these disruptions are also visible in clinical settings, where clinicians have begun to notice higher rates of cancellations even for documented clients.

As we sat in his office, painted in calming colors with a fountain running in the background, I asked Dr. Arias how his clinic responded to the increasing number of patients failing to come in for appointments. "It was a rude awakening," he responded. "We had to implement business policies we never had to implement before, which are more consistent with physical and general practitioners than mental health practitioners, and specifically I'm talking about overbooking." Rather than filling one appointment with one client, Dr. Arias explained that now more than one client would be booked for the same appointment. "You know when you go to your primary care physician that there are six people for that hour or four people for 11:15?" he asked. "That's because there are four rooms and they're counting on somebody not showing up. Well, our business is a little different. Our appointment is an hour and if you don't show up then I'm sucking wind for an hour." As the no-show rates increased, Dr. Arias noted that he and other counselors changed how they booked appointments. "We ask for five appointments a day for our counselors, and at least some time for some supervision and note writing. So we started making appointments for seven or eight people just so that we can net five. That's a business practice we never had to do before."

In addition to overbooking, Dr. Arias explained he also had to change services offered for children and train staff in a new billing procedure as a result of HB 87 changes. "Because of these policies we changed how we're able to serve children. If a kid didn't have Medicaid or if the kid didn't have a CMO [care management organization], we could bill our grant funding," Dr. Arias explained.[6] "The policies that took place at the state level have required that now before we access grant funding we have to find out why this child is not in Medicaid or CMO and we need to do everything in our power to get them signed up for Medicaid or a CMO." This change resulted in Dr. Arias needing to train staff in enrollment procedures. "We had to train our intake staff to help families sign up for Medicaid, whereas we didn't have to do that before." Ultimately this process delays treatment for child patients, Dr. Arias noted. "Now we can't begin services for 30 days so we have to be putting patients on hold while we try to enroll people in Medicaid. And the reasons why they're not in Medicaid or CMO are several. There may be some confusion, the family had a bad experience, or they never did the paperwork because they didn't know or they were afraid, whatever."

Dr. Arias's need to overbook his providers is necessitated by an aggressive immigration regime that attempts to govern immigrants through fear. This specific practice fits into a larger framework of medical surveillance and imposing neoliberal governmentality over medical practice. Anthropologists have described how health providers and clinics can be entangled in legislative efforts to ensure complicity with neoliberal, market-based health care initiatives that promote individual responsibility for health care and shrink the role of the state in providing basic health and social services (Rylko-Bauer and Farmer 2002; Maskovsky 2000). New licensing requirements for providers (and all other licensed professionals) and criminalizing types of care provided indicate a type of control and surveillance of medical professionals expressed through immigration laws. This type of control specifically advances neoliberal forms of governance because immigration legislation may create scenarios in which providers must adopt new practices common in market-based medicine. As Dr. Arias explained, immigrant policing has increased the number of no-show patients at his clinic, which led his organization to adopt practices common in other settings, such as overbooking timeslots to ensure there is no financial loss for the organization. In other words, Dr. Arias had to become more entrenched in market-based medical practices because immigrant policing threatened the financial stability of his clinic.

Dr. Arias's response to laws like HB 87 demonstrates how immigration enforcement regimes work to manage providers' conformity with practices common in market-based medicine. Forcing complicity with neoliberal strategies in market-based medicine represents a more hidden form of provider control created through immigrant policing, concealed by more visible and overt strategies of control, such as requiring proof of legal status to renew professional licenses and managing potential patient populations by criminalizing certain types of care. To be clear, then, immigrant policing not only governs immigrants through fear but also governs health providers and requires that some providers adopt market-based strategies. Immigrant policing efforts aim to not only create an ideal neoliberal citizen among immigrants but also force some health providers into adopting neoliberal market strategies in their practices.

In addition to overbooking for appointments, providers at CETPA adopted additional strategies to respond to immigrant policing. Dr. Arias explained that some parents did not want to bring their children to CETPA's programs because they feared driving, like many of the immigrants described in chapter 3. As a result, CETPA purchased a small bus to pick up children from school and take them to the organization for intervention services such as counseling and mental health evaluations, tutoring, alcohol and drug abuse prevention programs, and other structured learning activities. The after-school youth program is housed in a separate facility inside a strip mall with several Latinx businesses, including a *botánica* (a store that sells traditional healing items), a café, and a salon. One of the children's prevention specialists, Carla, expanded on the necessity of the bus: "We have to provide them transportation because many of the parents are working and they have a big fear of driving, especially two years ago when the law changed and they were checking for licenses and they were doing stops, a lot of people stopped driving. They just completely stopped driving." Because they no longer drove, parents stopped bringing their children to her program. "They were bringing their kids to the program and they stopped because they were afraid to drive." With the bus, however, Carla noted, CETPA staff can collect the participants. "We pick up each of the students. All the parents have to do is pick them up from the program and take them home, so we are saving them one trip and it means a lot for them."

Like CETPA, another health-related organization providing services to undocumented immigrants in Atlanta changed service delivery strategies. A women's health organization that offers sexual health programs, abortions, and services for transgender, intersex, and nonbinary clients changed how it provided sexual and reproductive health information to Latinx women. The organization employs *promotoras* for an initiative aimed to improve Latinx women's sexual and reproductive health. One promotora noted, "People stopped coming to our programs because they were afraid of getting stopped by police." Her organization then changed how it operated. "So instead of waiting for them to come to us, now we go to them. We have sexual health education parties, teach people how to use condoms, talk about preventing pregnancy, all in people's houses. We have them invite friends, neighbors, their teenage kids, everybody." For staff at this organization, fear of driving dramatically reduced the number of participants in their sexual health education program designed for Latinx women, resulting in staff taking on a new burden of reaching out to community members and hosting events in their homes. "They know they're safe if they're at home and they don't have to drive, so we go to their houses."

DIFFERING OPINIONS

Although providers I met in Atlanta shared a perspective of resistance or described how immigrant policing negatively impacted their clinics, these perspectives do not reflect all providers' viewpoints. For example, at the state capitol one day, while I was preparing for a meeting with state legislators about HB 87, I encountered groups of graduating medical students taking pictures on the capitol steps. Near the steps, a few small clinics had set up tables with information about the services they provided. At one of the tables, I met a woman representing a Federally Qualified Health Center (FQHC) in north Georgia, near Dalton and the Tennessee-Georgia border. Renowned for producing rugs, carpet, and vinyl flooring, Dalton bills itself as the "carpet capital of the world" and is home to approximately 30,000 people, nearly half of whom are Latinx. When Minority Leader Stacey Abrams described some legislators' support for HB 87 as a way to shift blame for failed economic policies to immigrants, I immediately thought of Dalton. Between 2011 and 2012, the carpet mills in Dalton downsized, and as a result, 4,600 jobs were lost (Lohr 2012). Further, the "carpet capital of the world" is in Whitfield County, where the sheriff's office has a 287(g) agreement with federal authorities.

As the clinic manager from the FQHC and I began to talk, I explained my research and that I hoped to interview more providers, including providers at her clinic, if possible. At that point, the clinic manager explained that an interview would be hard to arrange but she wanted to share some concerns she had with "illegal immigrants" since we were "on the subject."

> It's just a huge problem for us. They all come in with fake social security numbers, or maybe it's a real one but they just pass it around. And we've discovered this because we'll look up a chart with the social security number and see the patient has lost 5 inches in height and gained 20 pounds since their last visit and uses a different name. And they get employer insurance! All those chicken plants and stuff, they give their employees insurance! They just choose not use [the insurance],

so they're coming to *our* clinic and using *our* resources because they don't want to use their insurance!

North Georgia is home to numerous chicken processing plants, most of which are east of Dalton, and it is highly unlikely any chicken plant provided undocumented immigrants insurance. Moreover, the clinic manager's comments indicate larger interactions among immigrant policing, labor practices, and health policy. As I explain in the following chapter, some of the immigrants seeking care from the FQHC in Dalton may have gone to hospitals and ultimately been sent away from them—a practice that, depending on the circumstances, can be referred to as "patient dumping." Furthermore, the types of identification that the clinic manager saw, which she claimed to be fraudulent, may be the result of a practice that anthropologist Sarah Horton (2016a, 2016b) describes as "identity loan." In her fieldwork with migrant farmworkers in California, Horton describes identity loan as a process where migrants use borrowed social security cards to work with the consent of the person from whom they are borrowed. The relationship can be mutually beneficial: the person "loaning" the social security number receives the benefit of collecting additional social security wages for later in life, while the person borrowing the card is able to get a job. In some circumstances, identity loan can be exploitative, and Horton describes instances where employers coerce employees to use social security information belonging to employers' family members, resulting in an economic benefit for the family members who "loaned" out their documentation. As Horton argues, such exploitative processes thrive because of requirements created through the Immigration Reform and Control Act (IRCA), which, as I described in chapter 1, requires employers to check the work authorization status of employees. This requirement, combined with the need for cheap labor, creates the thriving identity loan market.

Although the clinic manager viewed patients as fraudulently using identification and resources, she lacked a fuller understanding of the types of labor practices that may be associated with precarious immigration statuses. It is possible that the immigrants she encountered in her clinic were involved in a type of identity loan relationship in order to work and support themselves and their family members. Rather than seeing the totality of the situation, however, this clinic manager only saw individuals who were undeserving of sympathy and of health services. To her, then, immigrant policing regimes may be a desirable way of responding to a population she sees as deviant and criminal without examining the larger context behind the patients she encounters.

CONTAGIOUS CRIMINALITY

Examining how laws like HB 87 involve health providers in immigration enforcement efforts reveals how medical authority can be used in biopolitical efforts to reinforce undocumented immigrants' criminality. Immigrant policing efforts can attempt to leverage the authority associated with health professions to advance biopolitical agendas. Criminalizing specific types of care that providers can give to undocumented populations uses medical authority to assert undocumented immigrants' criminal status, demonstrating how, as Foucault discusses, "medicine is a power-knowledge that can be applied to both the body and the population . . . and it will therefore have both disciplinary and regulatory effects" (2003, 252). In this situation, criminalizing a type of care that providers offer to undocumented immigrants serves as a disciplinary technique to normalize immigrants' criminality, suggesting that their inherent criminality is so strong that it can be transferred to providers, making them criminal by association. Health providers can resist legislative efforts to make criminality an infectious agent, and should consider the ethics of any other forms of legislation that aim to make them "guilty by association."

As I have shown in this chapter, immigrant policing and biopolitical expressions of state power can pervade health care settings and impact undocumented immigrants and medical professionals. Health providers are not immune from the consequences of laws that target undocumented immigrants, but they nevertheless have the ability to use their professional authority to resist immigrant policing efforts. The consequences of immigrant policing are not limited to individual health providers, however. Just as immigrant policing directly shapes individual immigrants' conduct, interpersonal relationships, and providers' professional practices, it also impacts medical institutions, as I describe in the next chapter.

6 · PATIENT DUMPING, IMMIGRANT POLICING, AND HEALTH POLICY

Driving north on Interstate 75 (I-75) toward downtown Atlanta, one can see some of the city's most iconic buildings rise above the tree-lined highway punctuated with traffic signs and billboards. Along the corridor between the northern and southern connections of Interstate 85 (known as "the perimeter" to locals), drivers can observe signs of Atlanta's historical and financial significance, passing symbols for Olympic Park, billboards for Delta Airlines, and clear views of the Coca-Cola headquarters. Before reaching downtown exits for Martin Luther King Jr.'s birthplace and the Ebenezer Baptist Church, the main artery of the metropolitan area dramatically curves around Grady Memorial Hospital, at which point a sign reminds motorists that "Atlanta can't live without Grady." Founded in 1892, Grady has been touted as an integral part of Atlanta's identity (Dewan and Sack 2008). The hospital opened with a mission to serve the poor and was one of the only institutions to serve African Americans. Grady's cultural significance, however, has not spared it from the negative impacts of immigrant policing and several political challenges that have threatened the hospital's ability to remain open.

Neither Atlanta nor Georgia could "live without Grady," which is the largest public hospital in the state and sixth largest in the country (Gamble 2013a, 2013b). Such a reminder would not be necessary if it were not for the hospital's recent financial tumult that pushed the institution to the brink of closure. Like other safety net hospitals, Grady has a patient pool of mostly indigent uninsured patients or patients covered by Medicaid, the federal health program for low-income populations (Gamble 2013a; Wynn et al. 2002). While other hospitals can use private insurance reimbursement funds to offset low Medicaid reimbursement rates, less than 10 percent of Grady's patients have private insurance (Gamble 2013a). Further complicating Grady's financial stability are its funding sources; the hospital only receives governmental funding from the state and the two counties where

Atlanta is incorporated: Fulton and DeKalb,[1] even though two out of ten patients come from surrounding suburban counties such as Gwinnett or Cobb (Dewan and Sack 2008). Providing care to indigent patients but not receiving adequate funding from counties, the state, or private insurers ultimately led Grady to a breaking point. In 2007, after running a budgetary deficit for a decade, the hospital faced potential closure (Dewan and Sack 2008).

An intervention from some of Atlanta's wealthiest business leaders ultimately resuscitated the ailing hospital, but the root problems that threatened Grady's financial stability continued. These problems included other hospitals persistently dumping patients (sending patients from one hospital to another without properly stabilizing them) to Grady, and a lack of compensation for providing care to indigent patients who live outside Fulton and DeKalb Counties. Grady is one of the nation's largest safety net hospitals providing care to all indigent patients and not just immigrants, and what happens at Grady reveals weaknesses in the nation's overall medical safety net.

Safety net hospitals see patients regardless of their ability to pay, and provide a disproportionately large amount of care to vulnerable patients, relying on federal funding to do so. However, federal funds for providing care to vulnerable populations have decreased because of measures associated with the Patient Protection and Affordable Care Act (ACA). As I noted in chapter 1, a key feature of the ACA was expanding Medicaid eligibility from indigent populations to all populations. Since Medicaid expansion was assumed to occur in all states, the funding set aside to reimburse hospitals for providing care to the uninsured was dismantled with the ACA because the policy's drafters no longer saw it as necessary. However, not all states expanded Medicaid. In states that did not expand Medicaid, like Georgia, shrinking federal funding and a lack of a reimbursement system for treating indigent patients complicated where the most vulnerable patients could find health services and how those services were financed. These concerns have been largely absent from debates about the ACA, lawmakers' numerous efforts to repeal the law, and proposals to replace it.

In this chapter, I examine the hidden interactions between immigrant policing and health policy.[2] I describe how immigrant policing plays a role in patient dumping, and I argue that patient dumping to Grady results in the state and federal government subsidizing private hospitals in Atlanta. I further show how the politics surrounding the ACA have threatened Grady's ability to be compensated for indigent care, which suggests that the health safety net for undocumented immigrants is further shrinking. A shrinking safety net ultimately points to broader shortcomings in the U.S. public health system. Moreover, a diminished safety net system demonstrates how efforts to increase immigrant attrition threaten public health care for all patients. To understand how immigrant policing impacts hospitals, I first describe how patient dumping works in a variety of ways. I begin with the story of Miguel, a patient who had had an operation at a hospital in Gwinnett County but ultimately sought treatment from Grady.[3]

MIGUEL: A GWINNETT COUNTY PATIENT SEEKING CARE AT GRADY

Miguel lives in a suburban Gwinnett County neighborhood across the street from a large shopping center with a grocery store, restaurants, and small businesses including a nail salon and beauty supply store. When I arrived at his home for our interview, he was being dropped off by someone in a small SUV, and he greeted me in his driveway. "Come inside," he said, welcoming me into his home and sitting next to me on a cold tan leather couch.

Miguel came to Atlanta from Guatemala in 2004; he arrived in the United States without papers, crossing from Mexico and braving all of the associated dangers with clandestine border crossing, like kidnapping, robbery, extortion, and assault (De Leon 2015). He and his wife, Carmen, have two children, five and two years old. Before his two-year-old was born, Miguel worked in a chicken wings restaurant in the nearby suburb of Decatur and commuted from a northern suburb, Chamblee. Driving home from work one evening, he was stopped by police and arrested for driving without a license. After his arrest, Miguel decided to move and look for housing close to where he could work, taking a job in the shopping center across the street from his current neighborhood. "I used to drive a car, but now they put me on probation, so I could no longer do that. . . . I was arrested and [the police] took me to jail, so after that I knew that I didn't want to get a car. It's better to walk than drive, so I looked for a job close to home and worked close by."

I asked Miguel where he worked, wondering what he did since there were numerous small businesses in the shopping center. He then clarified that he was not working at the moment. "I used to work; now I don't because of the wound I have. But I used to work just across the street." I was puzzled by what Miguel meant regarding his wound; he appeared able-bodied and healthy. "The wound?" I inquired.

"Yes," Miguel answered, pointing to his head, which was covered by a knitted black skull cap. "So one day, on my day off, I went to get a few things for breakfast, but when I was coming back, crossing the street here [by the house], a car passed by me, hit me, and knocked me onto the ground." I looked at Miguel in disbelief, and he nodded. He continued his story and explained that being struck by a car left him in a state of confusion.

"They hit me, and I fell to the ground, and when I fell, I never knew who it was or how they hit me. I don't know if it was a drunk driver or what." After falling, Miguel went into a coma. "I woke up in the hospital, but I woke up about seven days after [it happened] and didn't know where I was. When someone falls like that they die because a blow to the head like that—nobody can recover from that kind of blow to the head, nobody can withstand it, so I didn't know anything." When Miguel woke from his weeklong coma, he was confused about his surroundings and unsure of who he was. "After it happened, I woke up, but I never understood what was happening and I couldn't talk."

For more than two weeks Miguel was surrounded by his loved ones, but he did not recognize them. "For about 15 days I couldn't really see who was around; my family was there with me, my wife was there, my two brothers, but I told them that I didn't know who they were because that was my understanding; the wound did that to me. I said 'who are these people? Who are you?' I didn't know they were my family." Eventually Miguel began to recognize his family members and began asking what happened to him. "When I started to recognize them, I said 'what happened to me yesterday?' and they told me, 'it wasn't yesterday. You've been in the hospital for almost two weeks.'" Miguel's family was unsure what had happened to him and explained to him how he arrived home.

"They told me 'we don't know what happened to you because you came home, walking, vomiting blood; blood coming out of your mouth, blood in your nose, blood coming out of your ears; dripping blood.'" Miguel showed me from the couch where he had gotten blood all over the house, starting with the area immediately by the front door, and resumed his story. "They told me, 'when you came home we were worried but never knew what happened to you; we never knew. All we knew was that you went to buy something.'"

Taking off his hat, Miguel revealed that a large percentage of his skull—as much as one-quarter of it—was missing, giving his head a sunken-in, crescent shape. "They've removed all of this," he said, drawing an imaginary circle around the large, concave portion of his head, starting at the top, moving down the center of his forehead, and over just above his eyebrow. "The operation was up to here," he said, as he gestured up toward the center of his head, which seemed to have been recently shaved and hair was starting to grow back. "Up to here they took this piece out of me! I don't have this piece of my skull, and right now I'm waiting for them to operate on this one day. I told you it was Monday [when we talked on the phone], but that's not going to happen."

When Miguel and I first spoke, we tried to find a day to meet that worked around a surgery he mentioned he needed. I was not aware that the surgery was to continue the series of operations he has had on his skull. Miguel told me that on the Sunday before we met, a staff member from Grady Memorial, where he was to have his operation, called him and told him that the portion of his skull that was missing was still at Gwinnett Medical Center, the hospital where he was first admitted for care. Gwinnett Medical Center would not relinquish the portion of his skull to Grady until Miguel paid his medical bill.

"I have no money to pay for that hospital [Gwinnett Medical Center], because I am not working and they want me to pay them," he explained. "I found the other hospital [Grady] that gives you a card. . . . They checked me—they check every-thing, lungs, bones, everything. And it's all cheap because I have my card to admit me to the hospital." The card Miguel referenced was a Grady Card—the identifi-cation card that Fulton and DeKalb residents receive that allows them to receive subsidized care. As mentioned in chapter 3, to receive a Grady Card, patients must prove Fulton or DeKalb County residency; and for subsidies or reduced-cost care, they must demonstrate financial need.

Concerned about how he would pay Gwinnett Medical Center, Miguel explained he had a hard time finding work in his condition. "If I go to whatever job and they say to me 'are you okay?' And I say 'yes,' they say, 'you don't have a skull!' Bosses don't want to give me a job because I am already an injured person. I can't work anymore with this injury." In addition to having a hard time finding work, Miguel has also lost his sense of smell and taste, and he explained that he cannot hear as well as he used to, but he is thankful that he can walk and speak. "Through the grace of God I'm like this because I have seen cases where some-one had a head injury smaller than this one and couldn't walk, but I can walk, I can talk, I can go to the store and buy something, I can pick up my kids."

The accident that left Miguel missing a sizable portion of his skull happened only five months before he and I met. Miguel's attempts to contact Gwinnett Med-ical Center often left him frustrated; he claimed to be on hold for two hours or longer waiting to speak to someone who spoke Spanish before giving up or need-ing to take care of his children. "I take care of the kids because my wife works now, and I can't stay on the phone if they're fighting or something," he explained. Overall, the frustration sometimes mounted and took a toll on Miguel. "Some-times I feel like a weight is over me. Sometimes I cry; if I cry, sometimes I start to cry hard because sometimes I see no way out. How am I going to get my bone? And then I start to pray and ask God to take this sadness from me and move on, and I'm okay."

I asked Miguel if he contacted law enforcement after his accident. "Well," he replied, "I called the police after two months, when I left the hospital. I told them what happened and I asked them to please investigate and they told me there was nothing they could do. The officer said 'we can't do anything.'" I then asked Miguel why the police told him there was nothing they could do, and he said it was because he did not see the vehicle that hit him. "I didn't see the license plate or anything." Similarly, the police were skeptical about Miguel's story. "They can't believe it. . . . I had a scratched leg but I'm walking, and I can see, and nothing else is wrong other than the pain I'm in and this problem with my head. Many people think that a blow to the head makes you an invalid forever and puts you in a vegetative state. They told me 'we can't do anything' and they didn't do anything other than fill out a report. But they never did anything."

Although Miguel was awake when he walked back to his home after being hit by the car, he fell into a coma in the ambulance that his brother called for him.

He had vague memories of receiving injections in the ambulance before slipping into the coma, and he heard that he had been rushed to surgery immediately upon arriving at Gwinnett Medical Center. As Miguel mentioned, Gwinnett Medical Center still had the large portion of his skull that was removed during the emergency operation after the accident. Miguel worried he may not be able to have the additional surgeries needed to restore his head to its full round shape if he had to pay his entire medical bill, and he had already paid large sums of money for procedures related to the accident, such as removing large staples in his head.

"Before, when they wanted to operate on me, I went to a neurosurgeon to take out the staples, and they called me and said, 'you have an appointment on this day and when you get here you have to pay $3,500 for the visit.' I had to pay it because I had nowhere to go, and these were metal hooks in my head. They hurt, they hurt, they hurt! I couldn't bear those, so I had to go." Borrowing money from his brother and friends in the area, Miguel raised the $3,500 he needed to pay for having the staples removed. "So I paid and I went to the neurosurgeon and I told him I'm in pain [where the staples were] and I had thought he put them there to support the wound, and he told me no, just that he forgot [to take them out]. He forgot them!" Shocked that the physician had left the metal hooks in his head, Miguel was also surprised by the cost of the surgery. "I had been putting up with this pain for almost two months, suffering with this, and when I paid the $3,500 all they did was take out the staples, and that was all. Then they told me 'for your other surgery you need to bring $3,800 more.'"

Miguel exhausted his ability to borrow from friends to pay for his surgeries. "For the operation to put the bone back in my head, they said '$3,800 is your balance, what you owe. Pay this and then we'll put the bone back in.' But where will I get that money? My brother already gave me $1,700, the friends we live with gave us $200 and $150, so after they said 'bring the other $3,800,' where will I get it? I don't have it."

When Miguel started talking to friends about his trouble with Gwinnett Medical Center, several of them told him he should go to Grady to see if there was anything that could be done about his situation. As a Gwinnett County resident, Miguel was not eligible for subsidized services at Grady. When Grady faced near-closure due to its financial crisis, the hospital initiated cost control measures that restricted services offered on a sliding scale to Fulton and DeKalb County residents (Pizzi 2009; Woolhouse 2004). As one Grady provider explained, "If you live in Fulton and DeKalb, Grady is your hospital—you can go to Grady for free or pay very little out of your pocket because you pay for it with your taxes. Grady is there to serve Fulton and DeKalb residents." Despite living in Gwinnett County, however, Miguel was able to receive treatment at Grady, which was likely because his situation was so unique that it provided a valuable teaching case for medical residents.

Grady is a teaching hospital and accepts patients like Miguel in order to train new providers from medical schools at Emory University and Morehouse College. As part of its medical education tradition, Grady accepts patients transferred from other hospitals if they might be useful teaching examples. One Grady provider explained that "Grady accepts some [patient] transfer stuff in a long tradition of the teaching hospitals accepting outside cases." A Grady provider clarified how this process worked. "The reason they would accept someone from Gwinnett is because Emory or Grady has more specialization and can do stuff that other people can't." Noting the practice was common and he personally had justified transfers as teaching cases, the provider explained that communication regarding the transfer typically occurs between physicians. "Their attending [physician] will call the Grady attending, and the Grady attending will say 'just send them' and what's going to happen is the Grady attending will justify this as a teaching case and will give the residents something to do, basically."[4] However, not all patients who end up at Grady from other hospitals are teaching cases. Providers from Grady noted that most of the patient transfers to Grady were violations of the Emergency Medical Treatment and Active Labor Act (EMTALA). These transfers possibly constituted patient dumping—sending a patient from one hospital to another without stabilizing an emergent condition (Smith 2010; Lee 2004). Although patient dumping is illegal, the practice persists, and hospitals like Grady unknowingly accept patients that other hospitals have dumped.

Although Miguel may not have been dumped from Gwinnett Medical Center, he explained that only Grady was willing to provide his operation without forcing him to pay a large sum of money. Gwinnett Medical Center staff's emphasis of how much Miguel would owe if he had his operation there aligned with providers' comments about informal versions of patient dumping that occurred by stressing patients' financial obligations to hospitals. In other words, patient dumping consists of a variety of practices that extend beyond statutory definitions to include various forms of coercion and pressuring patients to leave one hospital and seek treatment elsewhere. Immigrant policing regimes exacerbated these problems.

PATIENT DUMPING AT GRADY

Patient dumping at Grady is a contentious topic. Not all scholars, health providers, and hospital administrators would agree with the providers I spoke to who claimed patient dumping was a problem because the statutory definition refers to failure to treat an emergent condition. Accordingly, some scholars and providers might argue that sending a patient who lacked an emergent condition to another hospital is not technically patient dumping. Regardless of the legal definitions, however, Grady providers described how staff at hospitals in Atlanta have sent patients to Grady because of their inability to pay and assumptions about their immigration status. While such practices may not meet specific legal definitions, they are nevertheless de facto forms of patient dumping. Grady administrators and providers found patient dumping especially frustrating because facilities outside of DeKalb and Fulton counties sent patients to Grady, but those facilities and their local governments failed to contribute to Grady's funding.

One Grady board member explained that hospitals sending patients to Grady without providing funds to support their treatment was a large part of the hospital's previous financial troubles. "Out of 159 counties in Georgia, only Fulton and DeKalb pay into the hospital," the board member explained. "The money they contribute is to serve Fulton and DeKalb consumers. When Grady almost closed in 2007, we realized that there were patients coming from 138 counties and only two counties were contributing financially, so Grady had to start a rule [to restrict subsidized patient care]." The rule the board member referred to was the residency requirement for uninsured patients, which involved providing proof of Fulton or DeKalb residency in order to receive discounted medical services (Grady Health System, 2019.).[5] "So Grady instilled some registration procedures and some payment procedures," the board member noted. The new procedures and residency requirements for discounted care were aimed to reduce the number of patients coming from other counties who had already sought care in another facility. "One of the biggest culprits was Gwinnett," the board member explained. "Gwinnett Medical Center would just say 'go to Grady' and that way they [did not] have to serve the patient. So we went to Gwinnett and said 'we would love to take these patients, but you need to give us some money,' and Gwinnett said 'no.'"

One Grady administrator explained that some hospitals sent patients to Grady because of its reputation for treating indigent patients. "There's this perception if you're poor, uninsured, undocumented, whatever, then, oh, 'go to Grady.' That other hospitals don't have to treat you; that we're here for the poor and that's what we do," the administrator explained. "And we *are* here for the poor," he continued, "but everybody's gotta pay into that system for it to work, and these other counties and hospitals aren't paying in. We're the ones totally absorbing these costs." To this administrator, other hospitals needed to treat indigent patients rather than funnel them to Grady. Alternatively, counties could contribute to Grady's funding, or the state of Georgia could increase Grady's funding for patients.

Funding to Grady is provided in part through the federal Disproportionate Share Hospital (DSH) program, which provides financial support to hospitals that provide care to a disproportionately large indigent population compared with other hospitals. As I describe later in this chapter, states can earn extra revenue by exploiting the federal DSH program. Furthermore, county boards determine how much of the state funding to contribute to Grady, and contributions vary depending on the budgets Fulton and DeKalb Counties adopt. Overall, these conditions make Grady's budget precarious and subject to several political factors.

Absorbing the costs for treating a large number of the Atlanta area's poor patients but receiving ever-diminishing funding from just two counties led to Grady's fiscal problems. As metropolitan Atlanta comprises twenty-eight counties (Office of Management and Budget 2009), patients from Cobb, Gwinnett, Clayton, Rockdale, and other counties may potentially seek care from Grady. Moreover, Grady is the busiest Level I trauma center in the region (Grady Health System, 2018) and may see severe trauma patients from outside Fulton and DeKalb Counties. With its role in treating trauma patients and location in Atlanta where residents from multiple counties can seek services, multicounty or larger statewide funding to support Grady made logical sense to providers I interviewed. "Grady has been begging for a statewide system for a long time," one provider explained. "It would be happy to absorb these patients [from other counties] if it had the financial support that was going to Gwinnett County come to Grady, but Gwinnett County doesn't want to give up that financial support . . . but they also don't want to see their patients." To this provider, then, facilities in other counties received funding to see indigent patients but rather than treating all of them, staff at the facilities would send some patients to Grady.

In response to the patient dumping and funding constraints that pushed it to the brink of closure, Grady underwent an enormous organizational restructuring that resulted in transferring power and oversight of the hospital from a government-appointed board to a nonprofit corporation. The change sparked protest from civil rights leaders and patient advocates concerned that, among other things, such changes would harm indigent black patients who relied on the hospital for care (Blau 2013a). Similarly, when the hospital closed its outpatient dialysis center, patient advocate groups and immigrant rights organizations held protests outside the hospital to raise awareness about the Latinx patients harmed by Grady's cost-cutting moves (Blau 2013b). As I described in the previous chapter, the dialysis center closure resulted in fifty patients, nearly all undocumented, being medically repatriated to their countries of birth, placed in private, for-profit dialysis centers, or needing to seek care through the emergency room through a costly, inefficient process necessitated because of insufficient definitions of emergent conditions and undocumented immigrants' exclusion from health insurance programs (Kline 2018b; A. Miller 2011a, 2011b; Williams 2011a, 2011b).

Changes to the hospital's leadership, led by former Georgia-Pacific chair Pete Correll, resulted in private foundations and donors collectively contributing $250 million to Grady's coffers (Karkaria 2008; Blau 2013c).[6] Of the newly generated funding, $200 million came from the Robert W. Woodruff Foundation (Karkaria 2008; Blau 2013c), an Atlanta-area foundation named after a former Coca-Cola leader (Robert W. Woodruff Foundation 2014). Additional changes to the hospital included laying off hundreds of employees and closing community clinics.

The new leadership also found donors to build new treatment centers, such as a stroke and neuroscience center, to attract higher-paying insured patients (Blau 2013b). The result of the changes was Grady's financial solvency, pulling the institution out of a $60 million deficit and from owing $71 million to Emory and Morehouse medical schools, whose faculty staff the hospital (Blau 2013b). Financial solvency and donations from wealthy donors did not increase the amount of money the state or counties contributed to Grady, however, and operating support for the hospital continues to come directly from Fulton and DeKalb Counties.

Because Grady is tied to funding from Fulton and DeKalb Counties, its financial circumstances are directly related to other counties sending patients to the hospital for treatment. Several providers noted that sending patients to Grady often occurred through concealed practices. As one provider, Dr. Tobias, said, "They [providers at other hospitals] wouldn't do it formally, like sending a note that says 'go to Grady,' they just tell them 'get in your car and go to Grady. I know you've got this horrendous condition right now, you probably have appendicitis. Get in your car and go to Grady.'" When I asked why this hidden form of sending patients to Grady occurred, Dr. Tobias explained that for most hospitals there was an economic motivation to not treat uninsured patients, including undocumented immigrants.

> If you're an ER doc, imagine you're working a shift in Gwinnett, and this undocumented guy [comes in] with appendicitis. We have to operate on him; not instantly, but sometime in the very near future. You're not supposed to let the sun set on that, but they can try to call the surgeon on call, and the surgeon on call's first question is going to be "what kind of insurance does he have?" Every time. But you know of course the guy has no insurance, and so they'll say "send him to Grady."

Dr. Tobias continued to explain that in some cases, ER providers participate in patient dumping, and it may not be willingly but because the administration pressures them to provide services to patients with higher-paying insurance. "It won't be the hospital's policy to do that, but it will be the practical effect of what the ER docs have to deal with. And the ER doc hates to do that," Dr. Tobias explained. "Why should one ER transfer to another? It makes no sense. So if one ER wants to send the patient to another [ER], they don't call the hospital's admissions staff; you don't go have another ER doc waiting for the appointment and redo what you just did; that's just very bad practice." Because it is bad practice, Dr. Tobias explained that patient dumping occurs clandestinely. "So you can't tell a guy to 'hop in your car' and send copies of the lab reports [with him] to take to Grady, because then Grady is going to call back and be like 'what the hell? You guys saw this guy already.' So it's a secret, just hop in your car and just show up at

Grady." Eventually, however, the Grady physician may discover the patient had been sent from another hospital, as Dr. Tobias noted. "The patient might even say that they went to the other place and then you look in their lab history and you find out later that they had just come from the other hospital." The situation Dr. Tobias described revealed how patient dumping can occur through subtle pressure on providers to give care to patients with insurance, and since undocumented immigrants lack insurance, they may be more likely to be told to leave one hospital and go to Grady.

Just as some hospitals may instruct ER patients to go to Grady for their initial treatment, hospitals and providers may also instruct uninsured patients to go to Grady for follow-up care. Encouraging patients to go to Grady for continued treatment further demonstrates how patient dumping can occur in subtle ways. As one provider, Dr. Lukas explained, "It's become less overt, but it happens all the time. You go into the ER in Marietta and they put a splint on you and say you need to follow up with orthopedics in the week, and it used to be they would write on their prescription pad 'Go to Grady,' and the patient would show up here expecting follow-up care for the fracture." Adding to this, Dr. Lukas noted that some hospitals are less obvious in their recommendations for patients to seek follow-up care at Grady. "They may say, 'follow up with this orthopedist,' who they're unable to get in touch with for whatever reason. Maybe they aggressively don't give them an appointment, but a nurse or someone will say 'you know you can just go to Grady and they'll take care of it.'" Dr. Lukas, who also held an administrative position at Grady, noted that Grady began documenting cases of informal patient dumping. "We started documenting that stuff because it's illegal under EMTALA, but we get patients every single day who show up saying 'they told me I could come here.' That's been going on forever."

Similarly, a Grady provider, Dr. Nelson, explained that covert patient dumping occurs through creating obstructions to care for some patients and that some institutions will try to avoid appearing like they are violating EMTALA. "What you oftentimes get is, you know, [this approach like] 'we'll stabilize you and then also you need to follow up with Dr. X,' and then you go and see Dr. X and Dr. X says, 'oh that will be $1,000.' And you know, [the patient says] 'I don't have that kind of money.' And then the doctor says, 'well maybe you should consider going to Grady.'" Dr. Nelson's point underscores how staff and providers at some institutions will intentionally emphasize the financial pressures patients would encounter if they continued seeking care at the first facility, which will push patients to go to Grady for care. This situation, to me, sounded much like what Miguel described after visiting a provider to remove staples from his head. Dr. Nelson explained, "They'll say 'you could follow up with me but it will cost you a couple hundred bucks,' which of course the person doesn't have, 'or go to Grady.' So we will get some version of that every day basically." Another provider shared a similar point, indicating some intentionality behind pressuring patients to go to Grady.

"They'll say 'sure we'll see you, it'll cost you $500 to get in the door; by the way, they don't charge at Grady.' It's not documented but it happens all the time—every day, and it's not so direct."

In explaining why hospitals dumped patients to Grady, one provider, Dr. West, emphasized the financial justification of patient dumping. "You have to remember that hospitals and health care facilities are businesses. Most of them are run by business officials; they're run by MBAs, they're not run by physicians, and it all comes down to money," he explained. "I don't say that meaning that they're all greedy," Dr. West continued, "but your budget has to be in the black at some point or you quit paying the light bill. . . . Your profits live and die off of what comes in and out of that door." Accordingly, in a market-based medical system like the one in the United States, dumping undocumented immigrant patients, who are denied access to health insurance, fits into the financial logic that undergirds health care institutions.

SUBSIDIZING PRIVATE CARE

As anthropologist Jessica Mulligan (2016) has argued, U.S. hospitals like Grady have become subjected to financialization techniques, resulting in facilities being restructured into "investment centers" where profitability, cost containment, and asset management inform institutional operations.[7] In Atlanta, the increasing financialization of U.S. hospitals has led to Grady's restructuring and other hospitals finding ways to bend EMTALA and to subtly dump patients at Grady. Since private hospitals dump patients to Grady, the publicly funded hospital ultimately subsidizes private facilities. As other medical anthropologists have shown, safety net health centers in the United States can financially benefit private health enterprises. For example, Deborah Boehm (2005) has described how Federally Qualified Health Centers (FQHCs) in New Mexico subsidized Medicaid Managed Care (MMC) by taking patients who could have been seen by MMC providers, shifting costs from the private MMC organization to the federal government. Similarly, dumping patients to Grady shows how publicly funded safety net hospitals support private health care organizations.

Pressures to remain profitable—a consequence of the financialization of the U.S. hospital system—play a role in why some private facilities engage in patient dumping. Nevertheless, these pressures ultimately frustrate providers because patient dumping is an EMTALA violation and morally questionable. "We've started reporting it to our compliance officers," Dr. Manheim told me, sitting in his office at the hospital. "Over the past two weeks I had a couple of cases. . . . We had a lady with a nine-mm kidney stone; her kidneys were not going to work and they basically sent her from this other hospital saying 'you should go to Grady because you can't afford to pay,' and they had admitted her and operated on her and everything." Dr. Manheim noted that Grady would be forced to absorb the cost of the patient's operation even though the other hospital should have treated her. "That's money the hospital's not going to get back for that, and if you see them, that's an emergency. A nine-mm stone should not be discharged at all."

While Dr. Manheim explained that sending patients to Grady alone was not necessarily an EMTALA violation, not treating emergency conditions such as a nine-millimeter kidney stone violated his understanding of EMTALA. "To be fair, if you don't have insurance and you live in Fulton County and you go to a hospital and they say 'yes you should have this procedure done,' and it's not an emergency, and then they tell you to go to Grady, I think that's fair and appropriate because we are paid to take care of these patients while other hospitals may not be." When hospitals send patients to Grady that are not Fulton or DeKalb residents, or send ER patients that should have been treated first, Dr. Manheim explained that he considers this poor professional practice. "If you're from Gwinnett or Cobb and we don't have an agreement, which we don't, then you shouldn't [send patients to Grady]. Each county has some public health services, and most counties' are not robust. In Fulton and DeKalb we are it." Dr. Manheim turned to his computer and searched for a file. "Here's one case. So [here's] a psych patient [who's] at a different hospital, [for example]; the patient gets agitated and they call the police and the police bring the patient here from the other hospital's emergency department. This other case," Dr. Manheim said, scrolling down his screen, "is basically the same thing, psych patient that they brought here. They don't want to treat patients that won't pay them, so they send them to us," he said with indignation.

Although some hospitals may not want to treat indigent patients, EMTALA does not sufficiently stop some facilities from sending poor patients to Grady. As one provider explained, "Everybody's answer is 'you have to go to Grady,' but [the patient goes] to the [other hospital's] ER and they stabilize the emergency medical condition and then they determine the patient['s condition] is not acutely life-threatening. That is all that EMTALA requires you to do." This statutory requirement, then, potentially protects some hospitals from being accused of dumping patients to Grady because the statutory obligations refer only to what may be considered life-threatening, which is open to interpretation. EMTALA requirements, as this provider explained, were not necessarily medically meaningful. "The words are essentially that you have to stabilize and that is more of a legal term than it is a medical term."

EMTALA uses a "prudent layperson" standard for providers to assess their legal obligations in stabilizing a patient, but the law does not have requirements for care following stabilization (Lee 2004). Moreover, EMTALA does not have any appropriated funding, and if it required patient stabilization for all conditions without compensating hospitals, then medical facilities would ultimately take a financial loss. "EMTALA is a good idea generally speaking," one provider argued, "but there's no funding behind it. I don't think we would have nearly as many [EMTALA violations] if the hospitals knew they would get paid by the federal government for uncompensated care," he continued. "Doctors don't work for free. . . . [The federal government has] said you have to take care of these people but we're not going to pay for it." Accordingly, the U.S. market-based medical system contributes to the patient dumping problem that Grady staff and providers routinely see. Ambiguous EMTALA requirements and a lack of funding associated with the statute have also drawn attention to how hospitals may dump or involuntarily medically repatriate indigent undocumented immigrant patients (Smith 2010). While in Atlanta, I heard stories of immigrants being sent from various hospitals to Grady, and quickly learned how patient dumping was connected to immigrant policing.

PATIENT DUMPING AND IMMIGRANT POLICING: A LICENSE TO DISCRIMINATE

During a *comité popular* meeting, one of the members, Rosario, discussed a bill she had gotten in the mail from a private hospital she had visited several months before the comité meeting. "I had to go to the emergency room and I got a bill for $12,000," she exclaimed. "They keep sending me these bills saying 'you owe a fifth for anesthesiology, or this amount for emergency,' and I don't know what I'm supposed to pay. Right now, I'm just paying the emergency room bill and I hope that covers it. It's not easy [to figure this out]." She expressed frustration with the cost of her treatment and indicated that someone at the hospital suggested she seek care at Grady. "I told them I couldn't afford [the bill]—[the hospital] is supposed to help you! They sure helped me [said sarcastically]—they dropped my bill from $12,000 to $9,000! And then they told me to go to Grady."

Rosario's situation demonstrates a type of de facto patient dumping that can occur for undocumented immigrants. When she expressed that she was unable to afford the first hospital's bill, staff from that hospital directed her to Grady for follow-up care. Moreover, Grady staff described how immigrant patient dumping was directly related to other hospitals threatening patients with calling immigration authorities. Stoking immigrants' fears about deportation and encountering police, then, became a way in which some facilities would coercively dump patients to Grady.

A Grady staff member, Micaela, explained that Latinx immigrant patients from other counties routinely came to Grady. Micaela's role at Grady was nonmedical, but she regularly interacted with patients. She was sometimes given the task of telling patients they were ineligible for a Grady Card and that they must seek care at hospitals in the counties where they lived. "We are not getting any money from Cobb or Gwinnett County," she explained. "And we try to tell patients 'you need to go back to that county' and they say 'they won't take us, they are threatening us with immigration.'" Similarly, another Grady staff member recalled patients who had come to the hospital after being turned away from another facility. "We had a few cases where patients stated that they went to [another hospital in Atlanta] and they said 'go to Grady,' and the patient said 'no, we're here,' and the hospital said 'well, we will call immigration.' They will do things like that." Immigration threats, then, are ways for hospitals to encourage patients like Rosario to seek care at Grady, which exacerbates Grady's existing patient dumping problem.

Micaela noted she would occasionally contact other hospitals when patients told her that they threatened to call immigration authorities. "We even call the other hospitals, we call Gwinnett, we call Henry County, we call all the hospitals and say 'we have patients that are in your county and are your [residents] that you need to service.' And they are like 'no.'" When I asked Micaela how other hospitals can legally send immigrant patients to Grady, she explained how EMTALA's ambiguity about follow-up care allows for this practice. "They are saying 'if they come to our ER and if they are in an emergent state and then we see them, it doesn't mean that we have to continue to see them.' It's that follow-up." EMTALA's ambiguity, then, allowed hospitals to send patients to Grady for a variety of reasons, including on the basis of immigration status.

While ambiguity in EMTALA creates one pathway for sending patients from one hospital to Grady, immigrant policing regimes create another. Micaela explained that immigration enforcement laws like HB 87, Secure Communities, and 287(g) created a "license to discriminate" against Latinx immigrants. Such a license involved hospital staff exploiting undocumented Latinx immigrants' fears of deportation. "[The immigration laws] gave [a] license to people to mistreat immigrants and it was really directed at Latinos, *Mexicans*," Micaela told me. "So I think that created a feeling of a stamp of approval to discriminate; the government pushed credibility to discriminate, it's okay to discriminate, they're 'illegals,' they're 'aliens,' they're 'criminals.'" As Micaela explained, immigrant policing laws created a type of sanctioned discrimination that allowed for some facilities to justify patient dumping when patients were assumed to be undocumented.

Just as immigrant policing contributed to law enforcement officers racially profiling drivers and stopping anyone suspected of being undocumented, it also contributed to racial profiling in medical settings. This type of "clinical racism" expressed itself through profiling Latinx patients and by threatening them with a call to immigration authorities. The biopolitics of fear, then, entered medical settings and could be used as a tool to make people afraid to seek services in certain places. Immigration enforcement laws have permitted a type of discrimination that leverages immigrants' fears of encountering authorities and being deported. "I don't think the law itself did much, but the license it gave and the environment it created, it made people more fearful," Micaela reiterated.

Micaela noted that the license to discriminate against undocumented patients fit into a larger context of governing immigrants through fear and racial profiling. She had witnessed intensified immigrant policing practices and heard stories of police stopping patients as they left clinics. "Police used to wait for people across from the clinic," she explained. "They were looking to see how people got to the clinic—if they were driving. So if you were driving, of course, where's your driver's license, and of course if there is no driver's license then right there you are being picked up. Cobb County, where I live, basically everyone was being profiled." Other interviewees similarly described patrol cars waiting outside health facilities.

During my fieldwork, local business owners who operated storefronts next to a shuttered clinic in a shopping center described how immigration enforcement practices resulted in the clinic closing. At a strip mall in a southern Atlanta suburb known for aggressive immigrant policing, I spoke with Paola, who owned a *paletería* (popsicle shop), and Abril, who worked at a hair salon. The two of them talked about how aggressive immigrant policing resulted in businesses closing in the strip mall, including the clinic next to Paola's paletería. "They sit here and wait," Abril explained, pointing out the window of the paletería to show me a *patrulla* (police car) driving by. "Or they set up a *retén* right there at the corner." As we sat in her paletería, I lost count of the number of police cars that drove by. The shopping center had every sign of being a dead mall, which Abril said was the result of the constant supply of patrol cars in the area. "All these stores used to be full; now no one comes here." Gael, the owner of a grocery store and Mexican restaurant down the road, expressed similar sentiments. "The police here have cut into our business; I had to lay people off."

The dwindling business at the strip mall where Abril and Paola worked and at Gael's store was the result of frequent *patrullaje* (patrolling) that I have described throughout this book. Latinx business owners in other parts of Atlanta also described the negative consequences of frequent patrullaje, but the situation at the plaza where Paola and Abril worked highlights how police targeting one strip mall not only impacted businesses like restaurants and salons but also had the potential to affect clinics. The clinic next to Paola's paleteria may have closed its doors along with other storefronts because police routinely sat in the parking lot or stopped drivers on their way to the shopping center. These practices further limited the number of places where immigrants felt they could safely seek health services. Facing threats of calling immigration authorities at some hospitals and seeing patrol cars outside clinics ultimately resulted in Grady becoming a place that some immigrants felt was safe only in case of an emergency.

When Anita from the comité popular abruptly fell ill at her workplace—a luxury hotel in downtown Atlanta—her husband took her to Grady even though it was not the closest hospital to where they lived. "I was throwing up blood. Pure blood," Anita told me at a meeting. "I left work and I got on the MARTA [Metropolitan Atlanta Rapid Transit Authority, the limited rail and bus system in Atlanta] and I called my husband to pick me up. I don't remember much; I think a man helped me get off the MARTA when it was my stop, and my husband was there.

He took me to Grady." When I asked Anita why she went to Grady, she explained Grady would not ask her for a social security number to prove her immigration status, and that she was able to get a Grady Card as a DeKalb County resident. "I'm still making payments on my bill," she added.

Grady is able to finance services to patients like Anita and Miguel, and patients who are dumped from other hospitals, in part because it receives DSH funding. DSH funding may not be permanent, however, which would create a precarious situation for Grady and, by extension, for all of Atlanta. If patient dumping to Grady continues, if it is exacerbated by immigrant policing, and if DSH funds disappear, Grady may not have the ability to continue operating. In short, immigrant policing and health policy changes through the ACA interact in ways that have significant spillover effects.

DSH FUNDING CONCERNS RELATED TO THE ACA

As I noted in this chapter, DSH funding is used to reimburse hospitals that see large numbers of uninsured patients, and through the ACA and Medicaid expansion, the uninsured patient pool was expected to shrink, effectively eliminating the need for DSH. This logic, however, did not account for some states, such as Georgia, refusing to expand Medicaid, and that legal challenges to the ACA would result in states being permitted to deny the expansion.[8] Accordingly, the ACA assumed a shrinking pool of uninsured patients because they would be on Medicaid, but in states such as Georgia, this was not the case. Moreover, assumptions about the needs for DSH funding did not account for undocumented patients, who are ineligible to purchase private insurance in the health exchange marketplace created through the ACA. In the aggregate, DSH changes raised concerns for some Grady staff that the hospital would once again be on the brink of closure.

In a single year, Grady can provide up to $200 million worth of services in uncompensated care (Gamble 2013b). For many hospitals, the DSH program is an important way to balance uncompensated care, and the program supported approximately 30 percent of all uncompensated care in the United States in 2008 alone (Hsieh and Bazzoli 2012). Since the program's creation in 1981, DSH payments have grown and become a "lifeline" for large hospitals serving uninsured and indigent patients (Mechanic 2004), like Grady. State governments administer funding to hospitals like Grady and ultimately receive a reimbursement from the federal government through the DSH program. This reimbursement scheme results in some states misusing Medicaid funds for efforts other than providing patient care (Mechanic 2004; Coughlin and Liska 1997). For example, states could collect $10 million from a hospital through provider taxes, donations, or transfers and then provide $12 million in DSH payments to the hospital; the state would then receive a fifty percent match in DSH funds from the federal government, providing the state with $6 million (Mechanic 2004; Coughlin and Liska 1997). In this example, the state ultimately nets $4 million from the federal government (Coughlin and Liska 1997, 2) and can potentially use the funds in ways that do not necessarily relate to patient care.

Furthermore, DSH funds can ultimately go to hospitals that do not see large numbers of indigent patients, as some providers reported was the case in Atlanta. This was particularly frustrating for one provider who viewed DSH funds as a way to assist hospitals providing care for indigent populations but saw the funds benefiting hospitals that had lower numbers of indigent patients than hospitals like Grady. "DSH funds are supposed to help support hospitals like Grady," the provider explained, "but it goes through the state, and the state's very political, especially when it's a white, conservative state, and you're a poor, black patient in a hospital. In Georgia, they've sent the DSH money democratically to every hospital that can show it, so Northside [a hospital in suburban Fulton County] will get DSH money while Grady's the one providing the services [to more indigent populations]." As this provider noted, decision makers about hospital funding did not consider which facilities saw the most economically and socially disenfranchised groups.

DSH funds were to begin diminishing in fiscal year 2014 in anticipation of a smaller uninsured patient pool through expanded Medicaid coverage (Linehan 2013). The timeline for cuts got pushed back until 2018, however, because several states refused to expand Medicaid and thereby insure more people. Furthermore, DSH funding remains in limbo as the ACA continues to be debated at the time of writing this book, and repealing the ACA may result in deep cuts to the DSH program (America's Essential Hospitals 2017). Decreases in DSH funding that occur in tandem with Medicaid expansion may disproportionately have negative impacts on undocumented Latinx patients and hospitals providing care to them (Castañeda and Melo 2014). Since undocumented immigrants are not eligible for health insurance created through Medicaid expansion (Kenney and Huntress 2012), they ultimately remain an uninsured patient population, and if DSH funds continue to be diminished, hospitals like Grady will no longer receive funding to reimburse them for otherwise uncompensated care. One member of the Grady board of directors was especially worried about this. "Right now, as it stands, I am very concerned about undocumented adults once the ACA is fully implemented. I've not seen potential sources of funding for the population. They've got nowhere else to go and are not eligible for Medicaid, and there's not going to be a billing source," he said. Similarly, if the ACA is repealed or eliminated through court challenges and DSH funds diminish, there will be few funds for hospitals like Grady to treat undocumented patients, who, in places like Atlanta, may be dumped to the hospital because immigration enforcement laws have created an environment of sanctioned discrimination that fuels unequal treatment.

For one provider who also served as a Grady administrator, shrinking DSH funds raised questions about the hospital's financial stability. "It'll be disastrous," he explained, adding that Grady's financial concerns are only part of his worries: "There's nowhere else low-income patients, including undocumented immigrants, can go. . . . I mean you can get cheap cash over-the-barrel health services for all kinds of people . . . but they can't do with anything that's beyond just a routine visit." Echoing this administrator, one provider, Dr. Arias, noted problems with Georgia governor Nathan Deal not expanding Medicaid for documented and undocumented immigrants alike:

> If you're a lawful permanent resident, then you have to wait five years before the Medicaid. That rule goes away if the state extends Medicaid under the ACA. . . . If Georgia doesn't expand Medicaid then you're going to have documented immigrants that don't have access to care. And then that leaves the undocumented immigrants in worse shape because before there were dollars available for uninsured people that included undocumented people [DSH funds]. This has gone away to pay for Medicaid expansion, and if Georgia doesn't expand Medicaid, then there are no dollars for the undocumented who don't qualify for Medicaid and no Medicaid payment available for the documented immigrants. So you're creating this bigger pool of people that won't have access to any kind of service.

Adding to Dr. Arias's concerns about reductions in DSH funding and not expanding Medicaid, another provider-administrator, Dr. Holt, feared Grady would not be able to stay open. "Grady can really be pinched [because of DSH funding cuts] and we don't have access to other funds through expanding Medicaid." Fearing the worst, Dr. Holt continued, "I mean it's going to be places like this that will have to close their doors because it's about $100 million or $200 million that comes in to Grady from that fund, and we couldn't operate without that."

EVISCERATING THE SAFETY NET THROUGH A "SLOW DEATH BY ATTRITION"

Decreased DSH funding and continued patient dumping may strain Grady, but other hospitals will also be impacted by converging health and immigration policies. One Grady administrator in particular noted how rural hospitals especially may suffer from decreased DSH funding, which may further strain the entire health care system in the Atlanta area. "If the DSH money goes away from Grady that's a big thing, but if it goes away from the rural hospitals, a lot of the rural hospitals, it's a huge thing. Some of them may close," the administrator explained. "A lot of them may close, including the ones where a lot of undocumented citizens in the southern part of the state who do a lot of the farming and all that kind of stuff are." Grady officials have publicly described how smaller hospitals may not survive DSH funding cuts and no Medicaid expansion in Georgia, and how Grady may have to cut services (Blau 2013c). If rural hospitals close and undocumented immigrants in rural Georgia are unable to access care, the administrator I spoke with thought it was more likely that patients would delay seeking care, which would have implications for Grady. "There've been two hospitals that have closed in the last couple of months, really small hospitals in Georgia, and there's a theory that there may be as many as 15 of them closing if the DSH funding goes away."

Considering the implications of fifteen hospitals closing, this administrator suggested that Grady could suffer from having to take care of a sicker patient group that is costlier to treat because they had nowhere else to go for care. "They are all critical access hospitals, you know 25–50 bed small area hospitals with quite honestly white poor, black poor, and Hispanic poor—that's who's served by that pocket. So now, with the hospitals closed, more likely the patients will just wait until the last minute before going somewhere." Waiting to the last minute will ultimately result in worsened health conditions, the provider noted. "That's more likely what you'll see; like they won't come up here because their stomach hurts, but they'll come up here because the mass that they didn't take care of, you know a big mass or something, that's what you'll see. And we'll have to deal with it, potentially putting a bigger strain on us." The strain on Grady, however, will be because of a politically created situation to not invest in health care for people living in the United States.

Losing DSH funding would ultimately contribute to inadequate care for all indigent patients in Atlanta, as one provider, Dr. Williams explained. "[Inadequate funding] causes long waits, so if you've got finite resources and a growing population, that means poor quality care, intermittent care, people who can't wait to get their medications, can't get into clinics for months and months and months, so, you know, they eventually die off." The eventual "dying off" is an unnoticed form of death and negligence according to this provider. "It's sort of a nondramatic, slow attrition, but it just means the quality of what we deliver gets poorer and poorer. . . . The trend is concierge medicine or boutique medicine for people who can afford it. . . . If you can't pay at all, then you wait longer and you get diseases of neglect and things you shouldn't be seeing in a first-world country." In other words, decreasing DSH funds would result in hidden but significant consequences for all patients in the Atlanta area.

Adding to concerns over Grady continuing to see indigent patients in its ER while other hospitals do not, one provider explained that some hospitals are restructuring their institutions to effectively select their patient populations, freeing them of EMTALA stabilization requirements by removing ERs and no longer having to take indigent patients. "A lot of hospitals have moved away from having an ER at all," this provider said. "They just don't have it anymore because sometimes the ER is just not profitable. . . . If you don't have an ER you can sort of select your patient population, people who want elective surgery and are not really that sick but are people who can cost a lot, I mean nobody is going to come in off the street." As this provider suggested, the increasing number of ERs closing is largely related to financial concerns, and between 1990 and 2008, 27 percent of nonrural ERs in the United States closed (Hsia, Kellermann, and Shen 2011). ER closures ultimately reduce access to care for indigent and uninsured patients while increasing patient burdens on other hospitals (Hsia, Kellermann, and Shen 2011); if national ER closure trends continue through Georgia, Grady may be faced with an even larger pool of uninsured patients than it currently sees but without adequate funding to treat them.

The impacts of potentially lost funding also extend to changing how Grady operates as a teaching hospital, as described by the provider who gave input on Miguel's situation. This provider explained that future cost control measures associated with the ACA may prohibit teaching cases from continuing. "Right now hospitals are running under tight margins. . . . Hospitals are just rabid with cost control right now. . . . More and more there is resistance to [accepting teaching cases]. The attending physician isn't the one that's going to resist it; it's the finance people who are monitoring transfers, so Grady is resisting that more than it has been in the past." The potential reduction of accepting patients like Miguel as teaching cases, combined with shrinking DSH funding and prohibitions on purchasing insurance through health exchanges, contributes to an increasingly limited ability for undocumented immigrants to receive emergency health services. This constriction in access will reduce the efficacy of an alleged medical safety net in the United States.

Although patient dumping, DSH funding changes, and concerns over providing uncompensated care for hospitals may not be overt elements of immigration enforcement regimes, they are nevertheless a component of immigrant policing as they complicate life for undocumented immigrants living in the United States. Immigration enforcement efforts collide with health policies to create new challenges for health facilities. Processes that threaten hospitals like Grady jeopardize one of the few access points undocumented immigrants have for care as they are key facilities in the broader medical safety net. When considered through a biopolitical lens, patient dumping, decreased DSH funding, and risks of closure for Grady and other safety net institutions, point to a form of managing life and death of an entire population.

The potential for decreased ability to receive care at safety net institutions demonstrates how changes to the health system through policies such as the ACA and practices such as patient dumping are ways of managing undocumented immigrants and *all* indigent patients. Challenges in providing care to indigent patients may result in patients eventually "dying off," as one provider explained, underscoring how health policies can be investments in life for some populations and simultaneously be a lack of investment in other lives. Although some forms of care for indigent patients, such as emergency care, are a biopoliti-cal exercise that can be an investment in life, they are insufficient, as Miguel's story indicates. Miguel's situation suggests how certain forms of health care pro-vided to some indigent patients are just enough to allow for survival but inade-quately respond to a traumatic health event, as evident in the large, missing por-tion of Miguel's skull.

Like the undocumented kidney failure patients I described in the previous chapter, Miguel, too, is left with a liminal form of life—alive and functioning but not able to fully live the way he used to, and unable to secure work in part because of the observable skeletal trauma he suffered. Miguel's body bears the signs of endeavors to manage life in the most basic of ways. This calculated form of barely managing life, or perhaps "mismanaging life," is codified by policies such as EMTALA that require not complete health care but simply the bare minimum: life stabilization in emergency situations. For patients like Miguel, who are vulnerable because of their immigration status, income, lack of health insurance, language ability, and race, rather than a full investment in their overall wellbeing, life stabi-lization is the only outcome they can hope for.

In this chapter, I have described how immigrant policing and health policy merge in unique ways and reveal weaknesses in the U.S. health care system. Just as immigrant policing efforts create a type of fear-based governance that shapes individual health behaviors, interpersonal relationships, and provider actions, they further merge with health policies and practices to reveal weaknesses in the U.S. medical system. Atlanta-area hospitals have a history of dumping patients to Grady, and immigrant policing efforts have created an environment of sanctioned discrimination against undocumented Latinx patients, as Micaela noted. This sanctioned discrimination translated to some hospitals threatening to call immi-gration authorities as a patient-dumping tactic. Such tactics would not be success-ful if it were not for the harsh immigrant policing regimes at work in Georgia that include, as Micaela described, stopping immigrant drivers as they leave clinics for care. Furthermore, if Grady continues to accept dumped patients, who arrive in increased numbers because of sanctioned discrimination, and if the funding source for treating those patients disappears, the institution will suffer, and by extension so will all indigent patients relying on it. Immigrant policing efforts therefore not only impact individuals, but through interacting with health policies, they also have implications on the overall medical safety net in the United States. In other words, the "slow death of attrition" one provider described impacts all people rely-ing on hospitals and is directly tied to immigration enforcement efforts that are designed to encourage immigrant attrition.

Sanctioned discrimination that exacerbates dumping undocumented Latinx immigrant patients from one facility to another, excluding undocumented immi-grants from health insurance, and police sitting outside clinics can all be chal-lenged. Moreover, the hidden consequences resulting from immigrant policing efforts interacting with health policies can be changed through action to advance immigrants' rights. As I show in the following chapter, immigrant rights groups and other activist organizations directly challenge immigrant policing efforts that place undocumented immigrants in detention facilities, lead to their deportation, and in some cases, result in family separation. These actions also serve as ways to combat immigrant policing efforts that have perpetuated racially informed types of patient dumping.

7 · "STAND UP, FIGHT BACK!"

On April 10, 2013, I joined the GLAHRiadores, other immigrant and civil rights groups, and more than 1,500 other protestors outside the steps of the Georgia capitol at a rally in support of immigration reform. From there, we marched through the streets of downtown Atlanta demanding an overhaul to the U.S. immigration system. After the march, civil rights leaders and local legislators spoke on the steps of the capitol and called for changes to federal immigration laws. Crowds cheered, chanted, and sang hopeful songs as Adelina and other local leaders pointed out that by closing down the streets and going to the Georgia capitol, legislators had no choice but to hear the protestors. The April 10 march was one of the largest marches GLAHR had organized. But both before and after that march, GLAHR organized numerous rallies, protests, and marches outside the Georgia statehouse, detention centers, and federal office buildings to draw attention to aggressive immigration regimes, including policies championed by the Trump administration, such as separating migrant parents from their children.

After the election of Donald Trump as president of the United States, GLAHR and other organizations joined a coalition to combat all forms of bigotry, including xenophobia, racism, sexism, and homophobia. Naming themselves the Georgia J20 Coalition after the January 20 inauguration day, the group comprises nearly thirty activist groups, faith-based organizations, and labor unions that sought to combat what they described as a "growing climate of hatred, bigotry, anti-black racism, Islamophobia, and xenophobia" (Georgia January 20th Coalition, n.d.). The coalition aims to "defend communities' human rights from a system rooted in income inequality, white supremacy, racism, and misogyny" (Georgia January 20th Coalition, n.d.). As part of this coalition, Adelina explained that she and the GLAHRiadores hoped to grow the number of allies for immigrants, encouraging members of the J20 to organize their own communities. "We want members of faith-based communities to organize their own networks and influence their legislators," she explained. In doing so, she hopes to expand GLAHR's immigrant rights message and reach new audiences. Furthermore, Adelina and GLAHRiadores have continued meeting with local police officers to discuss checkpoints in communities like Palomita's, which I described in chapter 3. Similarly, other organization leaders I met in Atlanta formed specific projects where they aimed to hold police accountable for their actions and challenge immigrant policing regimes.

In this final chapter, I describe some of the efforts immigrant rights organizations and other activist groups engaged in to challenge immigrant policing regimes and combat attempts to govern immigrants through fear. These actions complement the forms of activism I have already described, including *teatros* and marches, and fit into broader efforts to advance the rights of racial, sexual, and gender minorities. I also provide suggestions for what readers can do to combat immigrant policing and types of policies readers could pressure their legislators to support. Accordingly, readers who seek ways to disrupt the negative impacts of immigrant policing that I have described in this book can act against aggressive immigration enforcement and other forms of oppression by drawing inspiration from some of the activities described here.

STEWART DETENTION CENTER

One of the most disruptive consequences of immigrant policing is detention and deportation. The United States operates the world's largest immigrant detention system, which comprises more than 200 facilities and costs more than $2.6 billion annually to operate (Detention Watch Network, n.d.). One of the largest facilities, Stewart Detention Center, is located approximately two hours by car from Atlanta in the rural town of Lumpkin, Georgia. Lumpkin has fewer than 1,400 residents, and, as might be expected in an old southern town, it features a central town square where the city's courthouse sits, surrounded by shuttered businesses and the local police headquarters. The clean, beautifully restored courthouse stands tall, in stark, albeit shining, contrast to the vacant storefronts it faces in the center of one of Georgia's poorest counties. Visitors who walk or drive about one mile down Main Street to Holder Road will pass dilapidated houses and vacant land until they arrive at Stewart.

Like other detention facilities, Stewart is owned and operated by the private corporation CoreCivic, known until 2016 as Corrections Corporation of America (CCA). The facility was built as a maximum-security prison, which became apparent during my first visit. During that visit, as I approached the detention center, a water tower at the entrance greeted me with the message "Welcome to CCA Stewart Detention Center." Once parked in the asphalt lot where guards roamed and admonished visitors like me who tried to take photos, I approached a fence topped with barbed wire. When the gate to the outer fence opened, I stood waiting between the first fence and another fence, also with barbed wire. The barbed wire extended above the fence itself, up to about six feet high. The space between the two fences was still and devoid of life—there was no grass, and there were no weeds, just gravel that stretched until it met more fence and barbed wire.

Taking in my surroundings, I thought of the possibility of being stuck in the dead space with nowhere to go while both gates were closed. As I waited anxiously for the second gate to open, I talked to Tom, who had organized my visit to Stewart.

Tom and his wife, Karen, started an organization called El Refugio.[1] Located about one mile down the road from Stewart, El Refugio houses visitors to the detention center in its hospitality house—a necessity since Stewart holds immigrants from numerous states, and given the detention center's remote location, there are no nearby hotels. Detainees can easily get lonely; they can wait in Stewart for several years before being deported. "I try to visit folks as often as I can," Tom explained. "Some of them haven't seen their family in years." In addition to housing visitors, Tom also organized routine trips to Stewart with volunteers to speak with detainees whose family members were unable to visit them. Tom keeps a list of detainees, the languages they speak, and the last dates a volunteer visited them at El Refugio, or "the house," as he calls it. "The house" is an accurate description of El Refugio: it is a small, single-story home painted bright yellow, and had fallen into disrepair before Tom and Karen bought it to turn it into El Refugio. In December 2018, El Refugio expanded beyond the little yellow house when the television show, *Full Frontal with Samantha Bee,* donated a larger, six-bedroom house to the organization, expanding its capacity for housing family members visiting detainees (El Refugio, 2018).

Once Tom and I made it inside the detention center, we gave the guards our names and the names of the people we wished to visit. We then took seats in the crowded waiting area. "Now all we can do is wait," Tom said. Stewart's drab concrete walls were punctuated with posters extolling the benefits of private prisons and the need for good customer service. The posters, along with snack and soda vending machines and a lack of seating for all those waiting, made the detention center waiting area feel like a Department of Motor Vehicles office merged with the waiting room of a manufacturing conglomerate advertising to its visitors. The corporate posters hanging on the walls responded to critiques of CoreCivic and similar corporations. Despite the fact that detention centers are ostensibly not prisons, one poster read: "We all know that competition makes things better; why should it be any different with prisons?" Another asked: "Would you rather spend 11¢ a day on an inmate, or a second grader?" featuring a picture of a young, pigtailed girl holding an apple. Next to that poster, another poster assured its viewer that "those with a criminal history try to hide it. We make it public," a reference to the company running Stewart as a publicly traded, for-profit entity. The last poster I saw thanked guards for risking their personal safety by working in Core-Civic facilities, suggesting all detainees are violent.

During the hour that passed while we waited, we witnessed a security performance more times than I could count. In the waiting area, there was a folding table between an X-ray machine and a metal detector. All employees and visitors entering the facility had to pass through security, but the security procedures seemed arbitrary: some people had to take off their shoes before passing through the metal detector, and others were allowed to temporarily bypass the metal detector; some belongings were X-rayed while others were not. Most, if not all, of the security guards were black, prompting another researcher who accompanied Tom and me to comment on the racial realities of the facility, saying the detention center was a place where "white people hire black people to police brown people." The guards who entered the facility donned clear backpacks, white button-down shirts, blue pants, and combat boot–sneaker hybrids they removed when entering. The sneaker-boots, which extended to at least six inches above the ankle, seemed cumbersome to remove.

When it was time for us to go through security, we went through with relative ease and were taken through a set of double doors into a long hallway. From there, we were led to a nearby room with five small seating areas, each separated from another by half-walls of concrete cinder block. Detainees sat across from us behind a thick layer of glass, making communication possible only through the use of a telephone headset. There, I met Mateo, nodding to him through the thick bullet-proof glass separating us.

Mateo had been in Stewart for nearly one year. He was arrested in North Carolina after a dispute with a manager at a Piggly Wiggly store (a supermarket chain in the Southeast and Midwest United States). Before arriving at Stewart, Mateo was a soccer coach for a junior league team. He often stopped at the Piggly Wiggly on his way to and from soccer games, and one day he went to the store with his two sons, Fernando and Michael. During this shopping trip, Mateo went to use the restroom in the back of the store and left his two boys in the front, putting Fernando, the older of the two, in charge of Michael. While Mateo was in the restroom, Fernando ran to him and told him that Michael was stealing candy at the register. Mateo left the restroom and immediately went to discipline his son, but the manager of the store told him that Michael was never allowed to enter the store again.

Several weeks passed, and Mateo had to again stop at the Piggly Wiggly, but he was with Michael. It was cold outside, and Fernando was not with his father and brother that day, so there was no one to watch Michael if Mateo left him alone. Not wanting to leave his child unattended in a parking lot, Mateo decided to take Michael into the store with him despite the manager's warning. When Mateo walked into Piggly Wiggly with Michael, the manager's daughter recognized them and told Mateo he could not bring Michael into the store—he was forbidden from entering. Mateo got upset with the manager's daughter, explaining that no one could watch Michael. Pointing at her, Mateo asserted that "if anything were to happen to him, it would be your fault," and he left the store.

A few more weeks passed, and on his way to coach a game, Mateo again stopped at Piggly Wiggly because his eyes itched and he wanted to buy eyedrops. When he entered the store, he immediately got a box of eyedrops and went to the check-out line. While Mateo waited in line to check out, he realized that the box of eyedrops he picked was empty. He left the line, and when he returned with a new box of eyedrops, the manager of the store accused him of stealing. Mateo denied stealing anything, but the manager called the police. When the police arrived, they searched Mateo and they could not find the eyedrops, but they nevertheless arrested him because they suspected he was undocumented. He was sent to jail, and because the community he lived in participated in the Secure Communities program, his undocumented status was discovered. Without evidence of stealing, the state dropped its case for theft against Mateo. However, he was still processed for deportation and taken to Stewart.

While Mateo was in Stewart, his wife and children had not visited him; the cost of traveling from their hometown in North Carolina to rural Lumpkin prohibited them from seeing each other. As a detainee, Mateo worked at the facility as a groundskeeper and received a dollar a day for his labor. Other detainees worked in the kitchen and earned three dollars a day, but kitchen staff woke up at 3:00 A.M. or 4:00 A.M. to begin preparing meals, and he preferred not to work so early. More importantly, however, with his groundskeeping work, he could go outside and get fresh air. Though he preferred to work outside, Mateo was sunburned on his face and arms, which was not surprising since Stewart does not provide sunscreen to its detainees.

In a report prepared by the ACLU about conditions at Stewart, organization leaders described detainee abuse and neglect. Detainees are denied needed medical treatment for injuries and chronic diseases and are served nutritionally poor food that can exacerbate health conditions such as diabetes (American Civil Liberties Union Foundation of Georgia 2012). As Tom explained to me while we waited, some detainees receive only two meals a day, and some of them trade those meals for phone cards to call family members. Further, some detainees may not receive proper garments or bedding; in at least one case, a detainee reported being given soiled underwear belonging to someone else, which resulted in infection (American Civil Liberties Union Foundation of Georgia 2012). Detainee abuses in Stewart have even been fatal. In 2009, detainee Roberto Medina-Martinez died from medical neglect, and in public statements, ACLU of Georgia leaders suggested that deaths and abuses occurring at Stewart are because of CoreCivic's desire to cut back on services to enhance profitability. In July 2018, Efrain de La Rosa, a forty-year-old man born in Mexico, died after Stewart guards found him unresponsive. He was the eighth person to die in ICE custody in 2018 (Immigration and Customs Enforcement 2018).

As the largest private prison and detention company in the United States, CoreCivic manages more than sixty-five prisons and detention facilities throughout the country. Its revenue for 2015 was more than $1.7 billion (Nasdaq GlobalNewswire 2016), and CoreCivic is profitable in part because of its business model. The federal government pays CoreCivic and other private prison companies, such as the GEO group, a per-person fee for detainees. For such corporations, profits can soar higher by cutting corners, like reducing the number of meals detainees get or skimping on medical care. Cost-cutting efforts to increase profitability can result in unnecessary safety risks and reduced services to those held within the facilities, undermining efforts to humanely treat detainees (Anderson 2009). Such concerns were highlighted in a 2011 documentary, *Lost in Detention*, which focused on detention center abuses and brought to light the types of physical and sexual assault detainees encountered in a Texas facility. The film underscored that reporting such abuses might be met with threats of more abuse and neglect, potentially leading to death (Young 2011).

Being held in a detention center like Stewart has numerous mental and physical health implications. The facility does not have a doctor on-site, and in the event of an emergency, a detainee would be taken to the nearest hospital, which is forty-five minutes away. Without access to a physician, and with small living spaces holding numerous people, communicable diseases could potentially spread very easily, and chronic diseases may be difficult to manage. These conditions have prompted a series of activist challenges to how immigrants are treated in detention facilities, particularly at Stewart.

"SHUT STEWART DOWN" AND ACDC

Every year, activists associated with the Detention Watch Network (DWN) co-host a "Shut Stewart Down" event, where protestors gather to draw media attention to the abuses that happen at Stewart and other detention centers. DWN is a national organization that aims to abolish immigrant detention in the United States. As part of its work at the "Shut Stewart Down" event, DWN local affiliates provided telephone scripts to anyone willing to call legislators and vocally oppose inhumane treatment of detainees. Local affiliates also passed around petitions to sign and deliver to legislators, demanding an end to corporations like CoreCivic operating detention centers. The event typically starts outside the courthouse steps, where protestors convene and walk to the detention center.

At the 2012 "Shut Stewart Down" event, the GLAHRiadores and I met activists at the Lumpkin courthouse who had driven in from around the country. There, Anton, a leader from the Georgia Detention Watch group, gave a speech and described the route protestors would take to Stewart. He pointed out that the walk from the courthouse to Stewart would take everyone past the newly constructed sheriff's office, which he observed was likely built using revenue the town earned through its agreement with CoreCivic. He added that funds from the detention center also paid for the newly renovated courthouse that contrasts with the numerous dilapidated buildings in Lumpkin. Proceeding down Broad Street to view the new sheriff's office, we made our way to the detention center, quietly carrying banners and signs with messages opposing immigrant policing and detention center abuses.

When we arrived at the detention center, the entrance to the facility had been closed off by a gate, and behind the gate, several guards stood with their arms crossed, donning sunglasses and clothing with the CCA corporate logo. As a crowd, we gathered to listen to organization leaders, activists, and detainees' family members speak. Two women shared stories about having significant others in the facility. One of them explained feeling as if her family had been broken apart. A third woman who had been driving away from the detention center as we assembled at the gates stopped her car, joined the group, and gave a speech about her boyfriend, a PhD student at a Georgia university, who was in Stewart. He had told his girlfriend stories of abuses that routinely occur inside the facility. After these speakers, a man who had been detained at Stewart gave his account of what had happened to him in the facility, describing physical abuse, intimidation, malnourishment, and prohibition from recreational time. Leading a prayer for the guards who stood on the other side of the crowd that gathered at the facility, Anton expressed his hope that they would have a change of heart. As he spoke, the guards opened the gates for delivery trucks that approached the facility. "Commerce can pass through these gates, but conscience can't!" Anton exclaimed.

GLAHR also organized events similar to the Shut Stewart Down protest outside other detention facilities, such as the Atlanta City Detention Center (ACDC). At one protest outside of ACDC, GLAHRiadores and I joined the organizers of the undocubus, the group I described in chapter 4 that traveled across the country, stopping at major cities to host immigration rallies and vocalize demands for immigration reform. Carrying a banner with two members of the undocubus team, I joined the chorus of chants that we repeated as one GLAHRiador spoke them through a microphone. "Immigrants are under attack! What do we do? Stand up, fight back! What do we do? Stand up, fight back!" As we stood along the street holding banners and signs while chanting, ACDC officers filed out of the building and formed a semicircle on the top of the steps leading to the facility. Hands crossed in their uniforms and squared-off hats, they attempted to intimidate the protestors, perhaps fearing the protestors would try to forcefully enter the facility. In addition to the guards outside the detention center, patrol cars circled Peachtree Street while police officers stood across the street and farther down the block. After about thirty minutes of chanting, undocubus riders started a press conference and shared their stories about why they rode the bus to Washington, DC to hold a large demonstration for immigration reform. Among the undocubus riders, undocumented youth, commonly referred to as "Dreamers," made appeals for access to education, chanting "Education, not deportation!"

The ACDC rally and the Shut Stewart Down event point to ways in which individuals can vocalize and demonstrate their outrage with the kind of mistreatment that occurs in detention facilities. Protestors showed their continued dedication to challenging the abuses that occur in Stewart and ACDC, and publicly showed employees at the facilities that the actions occurring there were not universally supported. They further showed a refusal to accept the policies and practices that place immigrants in facilities like ACDC and Stewart. In addition to actions outside these facilities and marches at the capitol, activists in Atlanta also resisted immigrant policing regimes and racial profiling tactics by meeting with police officers directly.

COP WATCH AND ARTISTIC EXPRESSION

When police officers set up *retenes* outside Latinx neighborhoods and apartment complexes, GLAHR responded by holding meetings with local police chiefs and organizing marches from neighborhoods to precincts, as I described in chapter 3. Other organizations, such as the Cobb United for Change Coalition (CUCC), became frustrated with police for engaging in racial profiling tactics and began meeting with police to demand change. The CUCC members felt Cobb County police disproportionately targeted black and Latinx drivers, failed to respond to calls from black neighborhoods in a reasonable amount of time, and mistreated black residents. To combat these issues, the CUCC formed what it called a "cop watch" project, which involved CUCC members regularly meeting with police. For the first meeting with police, I joined the CUCC at the Cobb County Police Department in Marietta, a suburb north of Atlanta.

Passing through the glass doors of the Marietta station, I was greeted by a bronze sculpture of an officer, mounted on a rectangular pedestal, as if instead of a station I had accidentally wandered into a county police museum. To the left of the statue, a wide-but-short corridor led me to a wall of bank-style desks with multiple windows covered by thick plastic with round cutouts that allow visitors to talk to the officers on the other side. I informed an officer I was there to meet with the CUCC and the chief of police. The officer led me to a doorway, and I passed another police-themed artifact: a motorcycle mounted on a short platform. I followed the officer through the door and up a narrow, sharply turning staircase, eventually arriving in a conference room where CUCC members sat with the chief of police, John R. Houser.

The room comfortably accommodated the large conference table, where the chief and faced seven other people, including me. Joining the chief at the table were a captain and an assistant captain from another precinct. The conference room smelled like a guinea pig cage, and the walls were lined with wood paneling, adorned with framed pictures of old wooden bridges and what seemed to be late nineteenth- and early twentieth-century southern architecture.

Starting the meeting, one of the CUCC members, Sherlyn, mentioned her concerns with racial profiling. Sherlyn is black and lives in a predominantly black neighborhood, where residents assert police officers use a racial bias in determining whom they stop. The chief responded to Sherlyn by saying that he did not support or tolerate racial profiling. He added that everyone in his force gets trained in bias-based policing, and that Cobb County has a multicultural training block in its police academy, something other academies lack. As evidence of the police not engaging in racial profiling, the chief and the captain offered to show videos of police members being tased, since Taser use was a concern for Cobb County residents at one point. The captain alluded to this by saying: "I know you saw that YouTube video of a guy being tased and it sounded like we were beating the hell out of him, but as some of you saw on our videos, every officer who carries a Taser gets tased, and the sounds we made on our videos sound a lot like his."

The chief also claimed that he hires only "the best of the best" and that he would discipline anyone acting inappropriately. Sherlyn was not convinced, however, suggesting that police protect their own staff. "We write a complaint about a cop, who gives it to another cop to look into." The chief adamantly assured Sherlyn that he was willing to discipline and terminate any person on his force. Ensuring that his employees behave appropriately is why cruisers have been outfitted with video cameras, he added. "When I was an officer, no one was watching me and everyone was a sir or ma'am until they proved otherwise, but nowadays you have to watch people, and the cameras allow us to make sure our officers are treating everyone with respect." Sherlyn's concerns opened the conversation to discussing Latinx immigrants distrusting police officers, with one CUCC member, Joaquín, stating that Latinxs do not trust Cobb police because they fear being deported. Chief Houser responded by saying he had no interest in determining anyone's immigration status.

"You're confusing us with the sheriff," the chief said, referring to Cobb County sheriff Neil Warren, who on his website touts himself as "one of America's toughest [s]heriffs on illegal immigration." "We're not the sheriff—I couldn't care *less* about someone's immigration status. We just don't care. Our job is to protect Cobb—we're not immigration enforcement—we're too busy and we don't have the resources to do immigration work." One of the CUCC members interjected. "You're not the sheriff?" To which the chief replied, "No, and citizens get us confused so I'm sure immigrants do too, but the sheriff runs the jail and is elected. Our job is to protect the community."

It is unsurprising that CUCC members were confused about county police and the county sheriff. County police are relatively rare in the United States, but in Georgia, twelve counties have their own law enforcement agencies that exist alongside sheriffs and municipal police. County police answer to county governments, whereas sheriffs are elected officials who run jails and do not report to county government leaders. As elected officials, sheriffs in the United States are bound by state and federal constitutions, and their overall duties vary by county and state. The political nature of the position may also explain why some sheriffs attempt to cultivate an image they may feel appeals to voters. For example, Sheriff

Warren seemingly relishes having a reputation for targeting immigrants. He boasts on his website that he has been listed as one of the toughest sheriffs on "illegal immigration" (Cobb County Sheriff's Office 2015), and in 2018 he demanded that Congress defend ICE amid criticism of ICE officials at the border separating parents and children (*Marietta Daily Journal* 2018).

Further distancing himself from Neil Warren, the chief explained that the sheriff "may want to flex his muscles and seem tough," but Cobb County police have no interest in engaging in any type of immigration enforcement. He and the captain used a local activist, Amelia, as an example. "Amelia was here wearing [a shirt that said "undocumented and unafraid"] and we didn't care," he said, chuckling and referencing a meeting Amelia held with police several weeks earlier to express her concerns about racially profiling immigrants. The chief further deflected community members' concerns by pointing out that he was not Neil Warren and asserting he was not interested in anyone's immigration status. He continued to attempt to redirect the conversation, and after talking about officers not having raises for four years, the benefits of police departments doing community outreach programs, concerns for minor issues such as noise, and police departments not having ample funding, a CUCC member pressed on the issue of checkpoints.

"Let's talk about it now. Well, the checkpoints—what's going on with them? People see them and call in and text all over so we know what's happening." The chief, laughing, said, "I don't want to be on those texts," shifting his body language from being slightly reclined in his seat with his arms open to leaning further back with his arms closed. "You have cause for concern," he added, "but we're doing this for DUIs and things like that." The CUCC member added that he had lived in other states and had never seen a checkpoint before. At that moment I interjected, hoping to have police explain to me why they *do* have checkpoints. The chief leaned forward, hovering over the table as people all began to talk at once about the checkpoints.

"For my own benefit," I asked, "since I've only been here for about a month and have never heard of checkpoints, can you tell me what they are and what they're for?" The chief turned to me, still leaning over the conference table, talking over a CUCC member. "They're to check for driver's licenses, seat belts, DUIs." He returned to his reclined, cross-armed position and again claimed that the sheriff was the one behind aggressive policing. "The sheriff may try to get out there and do checkpoints and write tickets, but it's all showing off. He can't write tickets even though he likes to say he's the one policing Cobb County." After the chief's comment, a CUCC member explained that the Supreme Court has ruled checkpoints unconstitutional, and the chief said little else about the checkpoints but defended them as necessary. "But we can talk about that more, next time, since we've been here a while." The meeting ended with everyone shaking hands and thanking the chief, the captain, and the other officer for their time.

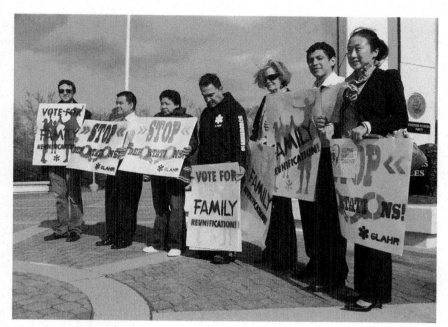

FIGURE 12. Holding family reunification signs outside a legislator's office during the "Keeping Families Together" bus tour. (Photo by Ponciano Ugalde.)

The CUCC effort to meet with police and express concerns was a way for CUCC to begin holding law enforcement agencies accountable for their actions. Similarly, GLAHRiadores and Adelina frequently met with police chiefs to demand an end to racial profiling. Such efforts resulted in some decreases in checkpoints, as Palomita described in chapter 3, and when the checkpoints increased, Adelina would organize follow-up meetings with police. A measurable effect of these efforts is hard to demonstrate, but such efforts signal to local police that community members are surveilling them and will question their actions.

Not all forms of resisting immigrant policing and broader forms of inequality take shape in police meetings, boycotts, protests outside government and corporate buildings, marches, or rallies (see figure 12). Instead, resistance efforts can also result in creative forms of protest. For example, one creative act of resistance GLAHR engaged in included a collaborative GLAHRte (a portmanteau of GLAHR and *arte*; see figure 13) exhibit in which GLAHR members and immigration activists displayed self-created artwork in a public gallery highlighting concerns facing immigrant communities. GLAHR members and I created papier-mâché birds that were installed around a large papier-mâché sun that GLAHRiadores created. Local artists and community members contributed to the exhibit with art that included overt political statements, such as images of the Statue of Liberty not welcoming Mexicans into the United States, and playful art

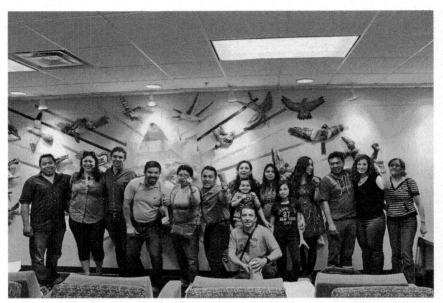

FIGURE 13. Papier-mâché birds and a sun at a GLAHRte exhibit. (Photo by Ponciano Ugalde.)

that included "undocu-valentines" and "undocu-pickup lines." "Undocu-pickup lines" included statements like "I'm no stranger to handcuffs" and "I'll drop the 'L' word [love] and the 'I' word [illegal] for you," playing with themes of policing, romance, sexuality, and commitment.[2]

GLAHRte and other creative expressions of activism, like the teatro popular events I described in chapter 4, underscore that resistance efforts can take a variety of forms and involve multiple types of expression that are not limited to holding banners or picket signs in large public spaces. In the aggregate, surveilling police through something like a cop watch project and using artistic expression to denounce aggressive policing regimes are ways to combat immigrant policing. Accordingly, I aim for readers of this book to consider how they might combat immigrant policing or other forms of oppression rooted in notions of difference.

THE BIGGER PICTURE: POLICING IMMIGRANTS, RACE, GENDER, AND SEXUAL ORIENTATION

CUCC's Cop Watch project, GLAHRte, GLAHR's meetings with police officers, and similar actions fit into broader activist efforts to confront law enforcement misconduct in the United States. Such confrontation is a way to fight against unjust legal systems and social inequalities that operate based on notions of human differences like race. For example, one of the most notable movements confronting police abuse in the United States, the Black Lives Matter movement, has specifically drawn attention to how police officers play a role in perpetuating racial injustice and how unarmed black men and women unjustly die from police officers' gunfire. As historian Russell Rickford (2016) argues, what started as a Twitter hashtag has become a critical activist network resisting police misconduct. The movement has provided persistent attention to how police practices, like stop-and-frisk, which entails officers detaining and questioning individuals, and policing theories like broken windows, which posits that vandalism and small crimes indicate more serious activity in a neighborhood, are ways to control and oppress black and brown bodies under a framework of criminality (Rickford 2016).

In addition to being attentive to police abuses, the Black Lives Matter movement has taken an intersectional approach to its activism. This perspective is demonstrated in its effort to "affirm the lives of Black queer and trans folks, disabled folks, undocumented folks, folks with records, women, and all Black lives along the gender spectrum" (Black Lives Matter, n.d.). Inclusion of advancing the rights of numerous groups in the Black Lives Matter movement exemplifies ways to avoid reproducing separations based on socially driven notions of difference. Further, this broad form of inclusion, as Rickford (2016) argues, has drawn attention to how oppressing black and queer lives fits into a nexus of state violence.

As I described in chapter 4, the U.S. criminal justice system has historically functioned to uphold racial power hierarchies, and law enforcement officers have played a crucial role in policing race. As legal scholars Joey Mogul, Andrea Ritchie, and Kay Whitlock argue, policing activities, law, and the U.S. criminal justice system reinforce racialized notions of difference, along with gendered expectations, and "predetermining who is intrinsically 'innocent' and who is blameworthy" (2011, 5:24). Some of the most salient examples of police officers being used to reinforce racial oppression can be drawn from civil rights protests in the 1960s. For example, when the civil rights activists the Freedom Riders arrived in Birmingham, Alabama, police officials agreed to withhold law enforcement intervention from stopping Ku Klux Klan members from violently beating activists (Arsenault 2006, 101). Two years later, public safety commissioner and white supremacist Bull Connor famously ordered police use of fire hoses and attack dogs against students who were engaged in nonviolent protest. Indeed, police have long been used to perpetuate racialized notions of difference.

Police compose only one element of upholding racial inequalities in the United States, however. As legal scholar Dorothy Roberts (2007) has argued, police terrorizing and targeting minority populations goes hand in hand with mass incarceration to ultimately maintain racial hierarchies. The consequences of racializing incarceration and police terror include political disenfranchisement and a loss of exclusion from full political citizenship (Roberts 2010; Uggen and Manza 2002). As Roberts argues, mass incarceration efforts targeting black men in the United States fit into a lineage of controlling African Americans that includes slavery and

Jim Crow systems (Roberts 2007; Wacquant 2001). Policing and the criminal justice system, then, can be used to assert and result in differential sets of rights and entitlements, and ultimately support white political hegemony. Immigrant policing efforts that culminate in detention and deportation are part of the broader apparatus of disenfranchising minorities through the U.S. legal system.

Political disenfranchisement resulting from incarceration and loss of voting rights demonstrates, as the legal scholar Michelle Alexander (2012) powerfully argues, how Jim Crow–era discrimination persists in a redesigned racial caste operating through a criminal justice system that sanctions discrimination against criminals. Immigrant policing fits squarely into this system since immigrant policing regimes arise out of efforts to govern immigrants through crime. The purported inherent criminality of undocumented immigrants may ultimately contribute to the abuse of immigrants in detention centers being overlooked or considered expected and appropriate for "criminal" others.

In addition to law enforcement being used to maintain racial inequalities, police officers also have been used to maintain gender norms and suppress LGBTQ+ rights. Officers have raided gay bars across the United States for decades, resulting in violence against LGBTQ+ patrons and arresting LGBTQ+ people simply for being in public spaces. Raids at bars such as the Stonewall Inn and Black Cat Tavern ultimately led to LGBTQ+ organizing and protesting police abuses (Branson-Potts 2017). These efforts gave rise to organizations such as Lambda Legal, which is dedicated to legal mobilization and advancing the legal rights of LGBTQ+ people. The work of Lambda Legal and similar organizations ultimately paved the way for rapidly overturning laws that targeted LGBTQ+ populations (Andersen 2009). Until 1990, homosexuality was a reason for being denied immigration into the United States and a reason for deportation (Mogul, Ritchie, and Whitlock 2011, 36–38); before 2003, same-sex sex was a crime,[3] and prior to 2015, same-sex marriage was prohibited at a federal level.[4] In short, legal mobilization around police abuses and legal inequalities has resulted in a number of legislative gains for LGBTQ+ groups.

Police activities that reinforce gendered and racial expectations do not exist separately, however, and often intersect. For example, in 2003, Detroit police officers raided the Power Plant, a bar frequented by black LGBTQ+ patrons, handcuffing and detaining bar patrons for up to twelve hours. Officers threw patrons against the wall, kicked them in the head, and verbally abused some of the 350 people in the bar (Mogul, Ritchie, and Whitlock 2011, 46). These and other examples of law enforcement violence against racial minorities and LGBTQ+ people demonstrate how, as some legal scholars have argued, "officers [have] used brute force to maintain raced, gendered, and heterosexual 'order'" (Mogul, Ritchie, and Whitlock 2011, 50). In other words, criminalization tactics have historically targeted LGBTQ+, nonwhite, and poor populations. Immigrant policing is another iteration of using law enforcement to maintain social inequalities by employing tactics like profiling.

HOW TO INTERVENE

Since immigration enforcement efforts operate based on understandings of racial difference and are related to ways in which law enforcement officers' involvement in regulating socially created markers of difference like race and gender, activists have an opportunity to unite and support one another's causes. To combat policies that advance biopolitical aims to divide and control populations, the best form of resistance may be to refuse to be divided. At many of the rallies, marches, and other events I attended while in Atlanta, protestors frequently chanted the popular song lyric of activism and unity I first heard in Georgia while driving with Adelina to the southern part of the state: "el pueblo unido, jamás será vencido!" (the people united will never be defeated—see figure 14). Indeed, if all groups and individuals who face various forms of inequality based on notions of social difference like sex, gender, race, sexual orientation, and ability were to unite, biopolitical mechanisms of control may cease to be effective. Accordingly, readers of this book can unite with organizations combating various forms of racial, economic, gender-based, and other types of social injustice to resist broad forms of control and efforts to maintain social inequality. In many ways, then, my hope is that readers will work to dismantle the many metaphorical walls that exist among people with differing immigration statuses, socioeconomic circumstances, racial and ethnic identities, abilities, gender expressions and identities, and sexual orientations.

More specifically, readers wanting to intervene in immigrant policing can take action to challenge aggressive immigration enforcement. An initial first step could be to participate in rallies, marches, political demonstrations, popular education efforts, and art and theater exhibits. By showing support, readers of this book can demonstrate a refusal to be complicit with immigrant policing efforts that disrupt immigrants' lives and communities and have ripple effects. Readers can also resist immigrant policing by finding local immigrant rights organizations like GLAHR or the undocubus movement and volunteering time, labor, or other resources. Further, readers can advocate for undocumented immigrants by dispelling myths about immigrants being drains on health and social service resources, especially because evidence points to the contrary.

In showing up to events, supporting organizations, and being an advocate, readers can effectively support the rights of all people, regardless of documentation status, to have quality health services, stable lives, and freedom from fear of incarceration, deportation, and separation from families, friends, and communities. Conversations about immigrants' rights and myriad social justice topics can be difficult, especially after the election of Donald Trump, who has vilified immigrants and social justice activists who resist white supremacist violence (Shear and Haberman 2017). Further, expressing opposition to xenophobia can be difficult when bloggers and internet trolls engage in a number of bullying tactics to challenge narratives that counter their opinions. Voicing strong opinions in

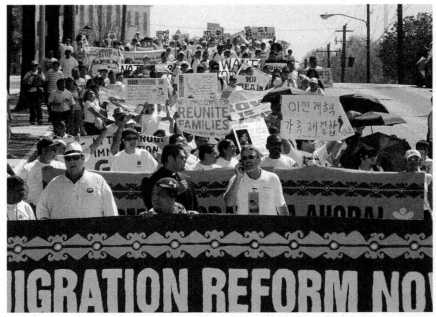

FIGURE 14. GLAHRiadores marching in downtown Atlanta. (Photo by Ponciano Ugalde.)

support of immigrants can be challenging, but these difficulties demonstrate the importance of countering rhetoric that reinforces racial difference and fuels social inequality.

In addition to engaging in dialogue, readers can take political action by contacting legislators about laws impacting immigrants. Following Donald Trump's presidential victory, authors of the Indivisible Project (2017) published a strategy online for constituents to learn best practices for reaching legislators and additional steps to inform political action. The section of the authors' guide that addresses how to contact legislators recommends that constituents have a specific ask for the member of Congress when making contact. If lawmakers introduce legislation that further aims to police immigrants, readers can contact their legislators directly and ask them not to support policy agendas that harm their communities and people living in them. Similarly, readers can contact members of Congress and directly ask them to support immigration reform that includes a pathway to citizenship, end Secure Communities, and end the 287(g) program. Contacting elected officials can be done simply through free text message–based services designed for political resistance like Resistbot, which will directly contact elected officials for users, craft emails, letters, and faxes based on users' text messages, and provide users with the phone numbers of elected officials' offices.[5]

POLICY RECOMMENDATIONS

In addition to taking individual action against immigrant policing, there are a number of needed policy changes that lawmakers could enact that would begin to address some of the problems I have described. When I first began writing this book, local and federal policy changes suggested political momentum to advance undocumented immigrants' rights had been growing, especially since GLAHR and the Georgia Not1More campaign actions resulted in sheriffs in some jurisdictions refusing to honor ICE hold requests (Redmon 2014; Georgia Latino Alliance for Human Rights 2014), and the Secure Communities program had officially ended (J. Johnson 2014). The election of Donald Trump, however, brought about a reversal of the progress that seemingly approached, demonstrating a need for robust immigration reform in the United States. Accordingly, readers should continue to advocate for long-term responses to improve immigrants' lives in ways that can outlast changing administrations.

One way to begin addressing some concerns would be to address federal exclusions from health insurance. The Patient Protection and Affordable Care Act (ACA) continues to exclude undocumented immigrants from health coverage, the effect of which, as anthropologist Sarah Horton has written, is that "undocumented immigrants will continue to remain dependent upon a fragmented and locally variable health care safety net for their care" (2014, 314). To address undocumented immigrants' lack of access to regular, primary health care, Horton suggests providing services and streams of reimbursement for care to undocumented immigrants, explaining that reducing undocumented immigrants' health disparities is a health equity effort in which everyone has a stake (2014, 315). Policy discussions about health care and the ACA continued after President Obama left office, and may continue for the foreseeable future. Accordingly, readers can engage in conversations about the ACA to assert undocumented immigrants' rights to participate in health insurance exchanges and be eligible for other reimbursement mechanisms like Medicaid.[6]

At a state level, state legislatures can and should enact policies that improve the lives of undocumented immigrants. Such policies include allowing undocumented immigrants to have driver's licenses and ending undocumented immigrants' exclusion from health and social services. California legislators, for example, proposed legislation seeking approval from the federal government to grant undocumented immigrants access to health insurance exchanges created through the ACA. Advocates of the bill noted that the change would save the legislature funds over time, since providing preventive care is more cost-effective than emergency care or other types of services; state officials, including Republicans and Governor Jerry Brown, supported the measure (Medina 2016). However, after the election of Donald Trump, legislators withdrew the petition, citing concerns about the new administration (Ibarra and Terhune 2017; J. Miller 2017). State legislatures, however, could continue efforts to permit all immigrants access to affordable health care. Further, as legal scholars have noted, federal efforts to prohibit states from doing so may be forms of federal overreach and directly conflict with states' abilities to govern the health and welfare of their populations (Gostin 2010; Kullgren 2003).

While state policies can have local impacts, federal policies are also needed to protect undocumented immigrants and end policing regimes that result in the deportations and detentions of immigrants who live and work in communities across the United States. One of the most immediate fixes could be a federal statute responding to driver's license exclusions. Everyone in the United States deserves the ability to be mobile, and with the lack of a robust public transportation network in most locations, driving is the only way for many people to lead their lives and complete necessary tasks like going to work, shopping for groceries, and being active members of their local community. Moreover, as public health scholars have shown, identification is needed for a growing number of daily activities, and policies that restrict government-issued identification impact immigrants' abilities to open bank accounts, cash checks, get a marriage license, obtain needed medications or see health providers, secure housing, and pick up children from school or day care (LeBrón et al. 2018).

In the short term, allowing undocumented immigrants to obtain driver's licenses would immediately reduce the number of arrests that can result in potential deportations. States control their licensing statutes, so readers can directly appeal to state legislators to change driver's license laws. Moreover, the federal government could mandate issuing driver's licenses regardless of immigration status by withholding portions of Department of Transportation (DOT) funding unless states comply with the requirements. Withholding DOT funding is within the purview of federal agencies through taxing and spending powers, and is how numerous public health measures are justified (Gostin 2008, 101); therefore, readers of this book can encourage state and federal lawmakers to address license issues.

The most important potential federal reform, however, is comprehensive immigration reform. Reform should include paths to citizenship for undocumented immigrants living in the country, regardless of age, and should not be intrinsically tied to economic factors. As anthropologist Ruth Gomberg-Muñoz (2016) has shown, currently there is no way for an undocumented person to easily regularize their immigration status, even if they marry a U.S. citizen. However, a wealthy person can easily become a U.S. citizen; through the EB-5 visa program, immigrants who invest a minimum of $500,000 can earn legal permanent resident status—a program Donald Trump has promised to keep while simultaneously promising to lower immigration levels (Patel 2016). In other words, wealthy people can buy their way into the United States, but immigrants who have built their lives in the country cannot stay. A federal solution to current immigration concerns must not reproduce inequalities or perpetuate existing policing regimes. Reform efforts must also not be prohibitively expensive and so exclude low-income groups, and must offer a permanent path to citizenship.

Immigrant rights groups such as GLAHR and the National Day Laborer Organizing Network (NDLON) have advocated ending 287(g) relationships and ceasing practices associated with Secure Communities. Similarly, GLAHR and NDLON have rallied for federal immigration reform that would grant amnesty to undocumented immigrants living in the United States and include options for family reunification of deported family members (National Day Laborer Organizing Network, n.d.).[7] The Immigration Policy Center (2013) has also supported federal amnesty programs as both a humanitarian and an economic stimulus effort. Readers of this book can support NDLON, GLAHR, and other organizations' efforts to end aggressive immigrant policing regimes.

Ending immigrant policing efforts must include opposition to efforts to further militarize the U.S.-Mexico border, as the border itself is implicated in immigrants' deaths. As Jason De León (2015) has shown, the "prevention through deterrence" program funnels migrants crossing into the United States from Mexico away from urban areas and into the Sonoran Desert. The program specifically exploits the landscape to end immigrants' lives as they attempt to enter the United States (De León 2015). Readers can oppose further militarization efforts, including proposals such as a fortified border wall that would perpetuate policies that result in deaths along the U.S.-Mexico border and in the deserts that straddle it.

While ceasing aggressive immigration enforcement policies is needed, so too is a way to respond to the long-term damage such policies have caused. Immigrant policing results in fear and trauma among some immigrants, and as anthropologist Linda Green (1999, 1994) has noted, fear can persist even in the absence of the conditions creating fear and result in lifelong trauma. The potential persistence of trauma suggests that the effects of fear may continue even if policy change occurs, underscoring how governing processes can outlive a specific practice or law. There must therefore be future efforts to reverse the potential implications of immigrant policing throughout the life course.

UNITED IN ACTIVISM

For readers who are students, faculty, or staff on a college campus, there are additional ways to resist immigrant policing efforts that constrain immigrants' ability to achieve goals like a college education. In Georgia, a group of university faculty and student activists, responding to the Board of Regents' ban on undocumented students from attending Georgia's Flagship universities, united and formed their own way to provide college instruction to undocumented immigrants. The underground education system, which they called Freedom University (or FU Georgia), provides free weekly classes near the University of Georgia. The university's name is a nod to similar historical movements in the United States. For example, when the U.S. Supreme Court ruled racial segregation in public schools was unconstitutional in the 1954 *Brown v. Board of Education* case, some school boards and universities were reluctant to integrate. In response, education activists organized informal education networks they called "freedom schools" (Blitzer 2017).

Classes offered through Freedom University provide University of Georgia–quality courses to students free of charge, and some faculty with Freedom University have mentored students by writing letters of recommendation for students to attend other institutions, including one GLAHRiador who ultimately received a full scholarship at a large university out of state. Following the Freedom University model, faculty, students, and other activists wanting to resist efforts to constrain immigrant rights can look to their own campuses as places of possible change. Potential activities could include creating programs like Freedom University or engaging in activities to make campus climates inclusive and welcoming of students with precarious immigration statuses.

Just as Freedom University shows resistance to immigrant policing, so can other actions on college campuses. For example, faculty and staff at the University of South Florida started an "undocu-ally" program, which provides skills to staff and faculty for supporting undocumented students, much like other ally models such as those for LGBTQ+ populations. Further, after Donald Trump's electoral victory, a group of anthropologists created an interest group of the American Anthropological Association that provides resources for how to support and protect undocumented students, sharing letters from the institutions that declared support for undocumented and Deferred Action for Childhood Arrivals (DACA) recipient students. Readers could look to these and similar resources for guidance on how to encourage their own institutions to issue statements of support, if they have not already done so. These and other efforts can help make institutions of higher education places that are free of immigrant policing and show all people the respect they deserve.

Professional organizations can also make specific policy statements and statements of opposition to immigrant policing. Health organizations, in particular, can lead the way in responding to immigrant policing. A growing body of research has demonstrated the health-related consequences of immigrant policing, including increased emotional distress (Hardy et al. 2012), mistreatment in clinical spaces (White et al. 2014), and inability or hesitance to use health services for which immigrants and their family members are eligible (Rhodes et al. 2015; Alexander and Fernandez 2014; Castañeda and Melo 2014). Immigration raids, in particular, can result in acutely high levels of stress and lower self-rated health scores (Lopez, Kruger et al. 2016). Data on immigration raids have also shown a relationship between raids and poor maternal health outcomes such as delivering low birth weight babies (Novak, Geronimus, and Martinez-Cardoso 2017). Mounting evidence directly implicates immigrant policing in poor health, and health-related professional organizations must continue to act counter to policies that have deleterious consequences.

Given the data on immigrant policing and health, organizations such as the American Public Health Association, the American Academy of Pediatrics, the American Congress of Obstetricians and Gynecologists, American Medical Association, American Nurses Association, and other health-related professional organizations have released immigration-related statements and can continue to condemn immigrant policing efforts. Health-related professional organizations could also prioritize immigration and health-related concerns through courses mandated by continuing education requirements and use their political influence to actively combat immigrant policing initiatives and oppose the privatization of detention facilities. Like professional organizations in the health sciences, organizations like the American Anthropological Association, the American Sociological Association, the American Bar Association, and others have taken stances against various forms of immigrant policing. Other professional organizations, including state bar associations, can adopt similar stances to reiterate the harms of immigrant policing and rally opposition to harmful immigration enforcement practices among members.

CONCLUSION

On the last Monday night meeting of GLAHR I attended before leaving Atlanta in June 2013, Adelina continued an ongoing conversation about immigration reform. When I was completing the research resulting in this book, President Barack Obama had won his second term in office, and among some immigrant rights activists, there was a sense that immigration reform was a possibility. Adelina, however, worried that any kind of reform effort that passed would exclude many undocumented immigrants, including people with prior removals and convictions. At the meeting, she explained to the GLAHRiadores the problem that possible reforms could create: "That will just make it worse for us because there will still be a large number of 'illegal' immigrants left, and then they will say 'what's wrong with you? Why didn't you fix your status the last time?' If we are going to have reform we need reform for everyone; we need amnesty for everyone, not just a few, but for all." Her passionate plea inspired head nods but filled the room with a sober sense of contemplation. "We have to continue to fight for amnesty for everyone, to stop breaking apart families and destroying our communities. We have to continue to fight."

Adelina's concerns underscored how policy can divide populations. Any proposed immigration reform that may continue to divide immigrants through exclusion criteria would effectively perpetuate social divisions based on immigration status. Adelina's fear was particularly prescient given immigration changes in both the Obama and Trump administrations. The Obama administration extended deferred action to some parents of U.S. citizens through the Deferred Action for Parents of Americans (DAPA), which provided temporary relief from deportation to a limited number of undocumented immigrants living in the United States with U.S. citizen children. This type of near-citizenship-by-proxy was an example of precisely what Adelina feared: an immigration reform with limited impact, resulting in ineligible immigrants remaining in precarious positions and perpetuating immigration status-related vulnerability. Moreover, as Adelina predicted, the precariousness of an administrative policy proved troublesome; DAPA faced court challenges that prevented it from moving forward during the Obama administration, and when Donald Trump took office, he rescinded the DAPA program and announced the end of DACA. After a series of court cases in 2018, the DACA program remains in effect, but its future is uncertain as some states, including Texas, Alabama, and South Carolina, are challenging the constitutionality of the law in federal court (N. Chavez 2018).

While DACA provides a reprieve from deportation, it is temporary and imperfect in that it does not grant recipients all rights and entitlements given to other groups of immigrants or citizens. Similar temporary programs like DAPA are also problematic in that they privilege undocumented immigrants with children, determining belonging partly by parenthood and raising U.S.-born children. Such policies uphold a heterosexual power regime and are not effective solutions for immigration concerns since they are underinclusive and reversible. The temporary nature of DACA and DAPA and their exclusions are nothing new, however. The United States has a long history of determining belonging based on white maleness, and restricting some Latinx immigrants' sets of rights on a temporary and renewable basis is another articulation of determining belonging, an echo of the ways in which nonwhite populations historically were restricted from full rights and citizenship. Accordingly, DAPA and DACA are additional examples of how, as critical race scholars have argued, the U.S. legal system supports and maintains social inequalities (Bell 1995b, 1995a; Delgado 1995; Freeman 1995). The Trump administration has further continued historical forms of privileging some immigrants over others, and has gone as far as to ban some immigrants from entering the United States at all (Gladstone and Sugiyama 2018). Through proposals to build a wall between the United States and Mexico, restrict authorized immigration to levels based on nineteenth-century statistics, and tie immigration to wealth, the Trump administration has created tiers of immigrant desirability not unlike those based on race and purported potential to become a public charge (Sainsbury 2006; Fairchild 2004), as I described earlier in this book. In response, readers can outwardly reject efforts to perpetuate policies that determine belonging based on heterosexist and racist frames, and efforts to govern immigrants through fear.

As I have illustrated in this book, aggressive immigration enforcement regimes create a form of fear-based governance that impacts undocumented immigrants' individual health, alter their interpersonal relationships, intervene in health providers' professional practice, and interact with health policies to threaten the stability of the entire medical safety net upon which all indigent patients rely. The numerous, often hidden, health-related consequences of immigrant policing necessitate action from activists, researchers, and the broader public. Challenging immigrant policing regimes will likely be a slow process, and as I noted at the beginning of this chapter, the calls to action and policy directions I have provided here are not exhaustive or meant to be prescriptive. Instead, the suggestions I have offered are a set of recommendations that I hope readers will grapple with and act on to improve the lives of immigrants who are routinely denied the rights and entitlements of other populations living in the United States.

ACKNOWLEDGMENTS

I am deeply indebted to a number of people who helped make this book a reality. I owe the greatest thanks to the Georgia Latino Alliance for Human Rights (GLAHR), and more specifically to the GLAHRiadores and Adelina Nicholls for their support, friendship, inspiration, and motivation. I am honored to have worked closely with social justice champions who welcomed me into their homes and taught me more than I can express. Thank you for all you do; *la lucha sigue*.

This book would not have been possible without insights from leaders and members of several organizations, including the American Civil Liberties Union of Georgia; Caminar Latino; the Center for Education, Treatment, and Prevention of Addiction; the Cobb United for Change Coalition; the Cobb Immigrant Rights Coalition; El Refugio; the Partnership Against Domestic Violence; the Feminist Women's Health Center; the Georgia Immigrant and Refugee Rights Coalition; Health Students Taking Action Together; the Hispanic Health Coalition; and Southerners on New Ground. Thank you to providers at AID Atlanta; DeKalb County Board of Health; Grady Memorial Hospital; Emory Healthcare; Fresenius Medical Care; Northside Hospital; and the Gwinnett, Newton, Rockdale County Health Departments for sharing insights with me.

I also owe significant thanks to the Anthropology Department and the Department of Community and Family Health at the University of South Florida, which supported the research that resulted in this book through fellowships and travel grants, and provided an environment that fostered my intellectual growth. I am especially appreciative for the years of advice and training from Heide Castañeda, whom I am fortunate to have as a mentor. Thank you to Angela Stuesse and Mathew Coleman, who included me on their National Science Foundation–funded study on immigration enforcement; without their support, and the funding from the NSF, the research resulting in this book would not have occurred. I also want to recognize Ellen Daley and Daniel Lende for their advice and guidance.

My colleagues and friends at Rollins College provided me an environment where I could complete this book, and I am grateful to be back at the institution that launched my passion for anthropology. Thank you to Bill Lopez for reading and providing feedback on several chapters, and to Laura Merrell, Erika Thompson, and the Salud team for being sources of inspiration and encouragement. My husband, David, who is an excellent copyeditor, read every chapter, provided feedback, and never lost patience with my needing to focus on writing. I am appreciative to have such a supportive person in my life who shares a commitment to social justice.

Thank you to the reviewers of this book and related journal articles for providing insights that ultimately led to a much richer understanding of immigrant policing. I also owe a great deal of thanks to Lenore Manderson for providing substantial feedback that strengthened this book and provided me with new perspectives for revising much of the manuscript. I appreciate the opportunity Lenore and Kimberly Guinta at Rutgers University Press have given me in being able to publish this work. Thank you for letting me share experiences about immigrant policing and provide ideas for how to stop unjust immigration systems that result in numerous forms of harm. *Adelante.*

NOTES

INTRODUCTION

1. The majority of names in this book are pseudonyms, but there are some exceptions, including Adelina. Adelina wanted her name and GLAHR's name to be used in the book. Similarly, I use Teodoro Maus's real name because he is a public figure and many of his comments can be found in publicly available sources like news media, including his comments about the 1996 Olympic Games. Similarly, in the following chapter, I refer to an incident involving a man named Rich and his dog, which can be found in local news sources. I also use Stacey Abrams's real name because she agreed to have it used, and I use the real names of officials sitting on the Immigration Enforcement Review Board. I also use the names of immigration critics like DA King when citing their public statements made in public hearings. Similarly, in the final chapter, I use Anton's real name because he spoke at a public event. Although I use the names of organizations and hospitals, I have made a point to conceal the identity of interviewees from those organizations.

2. Some readers may wonder why I use the term "Latinx" rather than "Latino/a." In using "Latinx," I am choosing to use a more gender-neutral term that is more inclusive of some immigrants' nonbinary gender identities. In quotations, however, I use the terms interviewees used, which was typically "Latino" or "Latina." Similarly, there are numerous ways to refer to immigrants in the United States who lack a recognized legal status, including "unauthorized," "undocumented," and "illegal"—the latter being an insulting and offensive term to many immigrants. I specifically use the term "undocumented" because it was the preferred term among interviewees. As one interviewee explained, "undocumented" captures the reality of their situation—that an arbitrary piece of paper somehow made people think of them as more or less than human, saying "It's like that fucking piece of paper is what makes me a human being, and it's like without that, I'm not a fucking human."

3. I use "Deep South" following a U.S. Census Bureau definition that has informed health-related scholarship such as Susan Reif, Kristin Lowe Geonnotti, and Kathryn Whetten, "HIV Infection and AIDS in the Deep South," *American Journal of Public Health* 96, no. 6 (2006): 970–973.

4. For more information, see Michael Hoefer, Nancy Rytina, and Bryan Baker, *Estimates of the Unauthorized Immigrant Population Residing in the United States: January 2011*, Department of Homeland Security Office of Immigration Statistics, 2012.

5. Outside of Florida.

6. There are a number of local parallels between Arizona and Georgia. In addition to Governor Nathan Deal campaigning on an Arizona-style immigration law, Cobb County and Gwinnett County sheriffs Neil Warren and Butch Conway have been reported to compare themselves to Maricopa County sheriff Joe Arpaio in local media and among activist groups.

7. The Eleventh Circuit Court of Appeals eventually overturned the provisions regarding assistance, but the rest of the law remains in place.

8. There are three models for 287(g): the jailhouse, task force, and hybrid models. The jailhouse model allows officers to inquire about the legal status of immigrants in their custody, while the task force model allows officers to inquire about immigrants' legal status while working in the field. As Capps et al. (2011, 15) note, this authority gives officers the ability to arrest for immigration violations and issue search warrants. The hybrid model combines the two approaches and allows the jailhouse and task force models to exist concurrently.

9. See the full list of jurisdictions with 287(g) agreements by checking: U.S. Immigration and Customs Enforcement. 2018. "Delegation of Immigration Authority Section 287(g) Immigration and Nationality Act." Last Modified 08/10/2018, accessed January 2019. https://www.ice.gov/287g.

10. These data were informed by two separate but related projects. The first was a research project to fulfill requirements of a PhD in applied anthropology. The second was a study funded by the National Science Foundation (NSF) that I worked on as a research assistant. As a research assistant for the NSF-funded project titled "The Devolution of Immigration Enforcement in the U.S. South and Its Impact on Newly Established Latino Communities" (Angela Stuesse, PhD, and Mathew Coleman, PhD), I conducted semi-structured interviews with undocumented immigrants, immigrant rights leaders, and others impacted by immigrant policing. Some participants were interviewed more than once. In this book, I primarily use data from the interviews that I conducted as part of my original PhD research, and I have drawn from NSF interviews to describe some informants' backgrounds.

11. The media analysis was done as part of my role as a research assistant on the NSF grant, and specific findings are not given space in this book. The media analysis served to triangulate interview findings and participant observation experiences and also provided an understanding of immigration rhetoric that helped inform research questions and data collection activities.

12. One activist thought it was important for me to meet Shirley Barnhart, who knew Martin Luther King, Jr. and fondly recalled her childhood crush on him. In many ways, this effort demonstrated how a shared political objective between a researcher and informants can allow anthropologists to have various types of engagement in a field site. These engagements require grappling with power and privilege, and as a white man I often reflected on the kinds of privileges I had when thinking about race and policing.

13. Some of the interview and participation observation experiences from chapters 3 and 5 can also be found in Kline (2017) and some of the interview and participant observation experiences in chapters 3 and 4 can be found in Kline (2018a).

14. Some elements of chapter 6 are derived in part from an in article accepted for publication in *Anthropology and Medicine*, titled "When Deservingness Policies Converge: US Immigration Enforcement, Health Reform, and Patient Dumping."

CHAPTER 1   HOW DID WE GET HERE?

1. The first order faced a number of legal challenges before being revoked and replaced by Executive Order 13780.

2. Indeed, in a polarizing move, Donald Trump pardoned Joe Arpaio for his conviction for criminal contempt of court, which was unusual both for the ramifications of the pardon and for the timing as the pardon predated Arpaio's sentencing for the offense.

3. Except for some Chinese immigrants in higher social positions.

4. The 1798 Alien Act, for example, allowed for deporting immigrants considered "a threat" to the nation.

5. Connections between biopolitics and anatomo-politics are best seen in institutions managing life, such as medicine, and when examining the foundation of contemporary disciplines concerned with population surveillance, such as demography and public health. Public health, in particular, is located at the very foundation of biopolitics—keeping populations alive, which can be seen in the heart of epidemiology and current governmental practices shaped by vital population statistics.

6. For more on "race war" discourse and logic, see L. McWhorter, *Racism and Sexual Oppression in Anglo-America: A Genealogy* (Bloomington: Indiana University Press, 2009).

7. Racialized policies have also impacted Arab-Muslims, leading to the racialization of terrorism suspects after the events of September 11, 2001. This has resulted in the deportation of hundreds of Arab-Muslim men from the United States, despite never being charged for conspiring to engage in terrorism, to appear as if progress were being made on the "war on terror" (Sheikh 2004). Policies targeting Arab-Muslim immigrants have had enduring consequences, as some evidence suggests that anti-Muslim violence and hate speech have increased in the past decade (Kretsedemas and Brotherton 2004, 11).

8. Undocumented agricultural workers could also receive primary care through migrant health centers, types of federally qualified health centers (FQHCs), as part of the Migrant Health Act. This is not to suggest that undocumented migrant agricultural workers had or continue to have adequate health services; on the contrary, undocumented migrant agricultural workers' health concerns are often connected to limited access to services, and all undocumented populations, compared with U.S. citizens, experience limited access to services.

9. The law also created requirements for employers to not hire or recruit undocumented workers. It further required undocumented immigrants who were being granted citizenship to pay fines, pay taxes, admit guilt, and demonstrate some knowledge about U.S. history and political processes.

10. Memorandums of agreement are also referred to as memorandums of understanding.

11. Although local jurisdictions have historically been authorized to enforce criminal immigration crimes, such as human trafficking or reentry after deportation, only the federal government had the authority to act on civil immigration violations, such as unlawful presence. MOAs created through 287(g) broaden local authorities' ability to enforce civil violations and blend federal and state enforcement activities. This is explained in an American Civil Liberties Union of North Carolina presentation by Katy Parker titled "Local Enforcement of Immigration—Secure Communities & 287(g). Furthermore, there are three models through which 287(g) works in practice: the jail enforcement model, task force model, and hybrid model. The jail enforcement model allows 287(g)-trained officers to question detainees about their immigration status and communicate findings to ICE (Capps et al. 2007). The task force model grants officers authority to inquire about immigration while conducting routine police activity (Capps et al. 2007). The hybrid model combines both programs in the same jurisdiction (Parker, n.d.).

12. See *Makowski v. Holder*, for example.

CHAPTER 2   INSIDE THE STATEHOUSE

1. The song was originally written by Sergio Ortega and Quilapayún and used to mobilize working-class people in Chile. The cover we listened to was by Inti Illimani.

2. Jim and all other names in this chapter—except for Stacey Abrams, John King, DA King, the IERB board members, and those who spoke at IERB—are pseudonyms to protect participants' identities, including other elected officials who requested their names not be used. As I explained in a note in the introduction, I use King and others' names when they attended public forums like IERB meetings. Similarly, I use John King's name as he is a public official who made comments at a public forum I attended.

3. Scholars such as Cindy Hahamovitch have also drawn parallels between sharecropping, slavery, and guest worker programs by describing how guest workers entered places with rigid Jim Crow laws and were sometimes subjected to harsh physical punishments. See, for example, Cindy Hahamovitch, "Creating Perfect Immigrants: Guestworkers of the World in Historical Perspective," *Labor History* 44, no. 1 (2003): 69–94.

4. Echoing Abrams, other legislators expressed similar ideas that Georgia's immigration laws, like HB 87, were in response to the federal government's failure to enforce federal immigration laws. One legislator in particular, however, pointed out the inconsistency with arguing that immigration was a federal issue and passing state-specific immigration statutes: "[Republicans] acknowledge that it's a federal issue, and I concur that it's a federal issue, and so then they go off the deep end and contradict themselves and they say 'we'll work and do something about it even though it's a federal issue, and we recognize it's a federal issue.'"

5. See, for example, Laura Nader's call to study powerful populations in L. Nader, "Up the Anthropologist—Perspectives Gained from Studying Up," in *Reinventing Anthropology*, ed. D. H. Hymes (New York: Pantheon Books, 1969), 284–311.

6. King publicly voiced support for the bill and posted Facebook messages on various anti-undocumented immigration groups' pages urging people to call legislators and voice support for HB 125.

CHAPTER 3 "WE LIVE HERE IN FEAR"

1. I have written about fear and immigrant policing elsewhere, and some immigrants' experiences in this chapter, such as Rosa's, first appeared in Kline (2017) and in Kline (2018a).

2. Elsewhere (Kline 2017), I have referred to this as a parallel medical system, but in some ways "parallel" might suggest equal, and for this reason I use the term "shadow medical system" here.

3. Angela Stuesse and Mathew Coleman have also written about Palomita. See Stuesse and Coleman (2014).

4. The name "Clínica Latina" is a pseudonym to protect the location of the actual clinic. Similarly, other names for clínicas and farmacaias are pseudonyms except for Clínica de la Mama since news stories can easily be found about the clinic's practices.

5. LEEP, or loop electrosurgical excision procedure, is one of the most common ways of treating cervical dysplasia.

CHAPTER 4   IMMIGRANT POLICING AND INTERPERSONAL RELATIONSHIPS

1. For more on Juan Carlos's story, see J. C. Guevara, A. Stuesse, and M. Coleman, "I Used to Believe in Justice," in *Forced Out and Fenced In: Immigration Tales from the Field*, ed. T. M. Golash-Boza (New York: Oxford University Press, 2018), 185–192.

2. For example, see the flowchart on page xii in Gomberg-Muñoz (2016).

3. For example, see scholarship on the Violence Against Women Act and its shortcomings for protecting undocumented immigrants (J. Abrams 2009; Conyers 2007; Davis 2004).

4. Several scholars have described how threats to call police play a role in gender-based partner violence. See, for example, Parson et al. (2016).

CHAPTER 5   "A DEATH BY A THOUSAND LITTLE CUTS"

1. This is a pseudonym for a faith-based clinic operating in Atlanta that sees immigrant patients. Although I use the real names of other organizations, I chose to use a pseudonym for this clinic because it does not explicitly advertise its services for immigrants and staff suggested a desire to not draw too much attention to the fact that they provide services to undocumented patients.

2. The cumulative number of providers affected was not reported.

3. Depending on the state, providers' warnings may be mandatory or permitted.

4. My description of the dialysis situation has been published in part in Kline 2018c.

5. This effort never materialized in any serious change, as the HHCGA experienced a complete turnover in staff and leadership that did not keep the efforts put in place by previous leaders.

6. Care management organizations are generally referred to as managed care organizations.

CHAPTER 6   PATIENT DUMPING, IMMIGRANT POLICING, AND HEALTH POLICY

1. The majority of the city is in Fulton County, with a small portion extending into DeKalb. The hospital also receives other funds from Medicare and Medicaid, some commercial funding, and some state funding for mental health and trauma.

2. This chapter is derived in part from an article titled "When Policies of Deservingness Converge: US Immigration Enforcement, Health Reform, and Patient Dumping," which was accepted for publication in *Anthropology and Medicine* © 2019 Informa UK Limited, trading as Taylor & Francis Group.

3. Miguel's story is also in N. Kline, "How Will I Get My Skull Back? The Embodied Consequences of Immigrant Policing," in *Forced Out and Fenced In: Immigration Tales from the Field*, ed. T. M. Golash-Boza (New York: Oxford University Press), 109–116. Here, however, his story is contextualized in a larger system of immigrant policing. His story will also appear in the *Anthropology and Medicine* article listed in note 2.

4. This situation may be more nuanced than this provider suggested. Another provider, who reviewed this chapter after it was drafted, noted that Grady will accept patients because "we have a high level of expertise and we have residents who can learn, but not for learning per se." In reconciling one provider referring to patients like Miguel as potential "teaching cases" and another provider saying that Grady accepts patients because providers have high levels of expertise and residents who can learn, I have decided to keep the "teaching case" terminology because it still reflects how patients will be admitted to Grady if experienced providers deem a situation worthy of needing expert care that residents may also learn from.

5. Unless the patient was accepted as a teaching case.

6. An administrator noted this figure was more like $325 million, but I could not find information to substantiate this claim.

7. I have discussed financialization related to Grady in greater detail in Kline 2018c.

8. When the ACA passed, Medicaid expansion was mandatory, but mandatory expansion was stricken because of the 2012 Supreme Court case *National Federation of Independent Business (NFIB) v. Sebelius*.

CHAPTER 7   "STAND UP, FIGHT BACK!"

1. Although El Refugio is the name of the actual organization, Tom and Karen are pseudonyms since their information is not made publicly available through the organization.

2. Similarly, in the wake of the Pulse club shooting in Orlando, Florida, which disproportionately impacted LGBTQ+ racial minorities, LGBTQ+ Latinx artists and activists turned to artistic expression to inspire activism and healing. Such efforts included art exhibits at local galleries and museums, and a mural installed at the University of Central Florida, where two victims had been students.

3. As decided in the *Lawrence v. Texas* case.

4. As decided in the *Obergefell v. Hodges* case.

5. Resistbot can be found online. Resistbot, n.d. https://resist.bot.

6. While advocating for increased access to health services is arguably being complicit with biomedical hegemony (see Lock and Nguyen [2010, 24–25]), I argue that medical anthropologists must challenge inequality and reduce the potential for disproportionate experiences of suffering.

7. Amnesty or legalization for all efforts has had increasing social media visibility through the #11MillionNow! Twitter feed and blog. See https://legalizationforall.wordpress.com.

BIBLIOGRAPHY

Abraham, Margaret. 2000. *Speaking the Unspeakable: Marital Violence among South Asian Immigrants in the United States*. New Brunswick, NJ: Rutgers University Press.

Abraído-Lanza, Ana F., Maria T. Chao, and Karen R. Flórez. 2005. "Do Healthy Behaviors Decline with Greater Acculturation? Implications for the Latino Mortality Paradox." *Social Science & Medicine* 61 (6): 1243–1255.

Abrams, Jamie R. 2009. "The Dual Purposes of the U Visa Thwarted in a Legislative Duel." *Saint Louis University Law Review* 29: 373–441.

Abrams, P. 1988. "Notes on the Difficulty of Studying the State (1977)." *Journal of Historical Sociology* 1 (1): 58–89.

Abrego, Leisy. 2008. "Legitimacy, Social Identity, and the Mobilization of Law: The Effects of Assembly Bill 540 on Undocumented Students in California." *Law & Social Inquiry* 33 (3): 709–734.

Aguilasocho, Edgar Ivan, David Rodwin, and Sameer M. Ashar. 2012. "Misplaced Priorities: The Failure of Secure Communities in Los Angeles County." UC Irvine School of Law Research Paper No. 2013-118. Social Science Research Network, February 8. https://papers.ssrn.com/sol3/papers.cfm?abstract_id=2012283.

Alexander, Michelle. 2012. *The New Jim Crow: Mass Incarceration in the Age of Colorblindness*. New York: New Press.

Alexander, William L., and Magdalena Fernandez. 2014. "Immigration Policing and Medical Care for Farmworkers: Uncertainties and Anxieties in the East Coast Migrant Stream." *North American Dialogue* 17 (1): 13–30.

American Civil Liberties Union Foundation of Georgia. 2012. *Prisoners of Profit: Immigrants and Detention in Georgia*. Atlanta. https://www.acluga.org/Prisoners_of_Profit.pdf.

American Nurses Association. 2010. *Nursing beyond Borders: Access to Health Care for Documented and Undocumented Immigrants Living in the US*. ANA Issue Brief: Information and Analysis on Topics Affecting Nurses, the Profession and Health Care. http://www.nursingworld.org/MainMenuCategories/Policy-Advocacy/Positions-and-Resolutions/Issue-Briefs/Access-to-care-for-immigrants.pdf.

America's Essential Hospitals. 2017. *ACA Replacement Must Protect Vulnerable People, Communities*. https://essentialhospitals.org/wp-content/uploads/2017/02/UCC-policy-brief-February-2017-FINAL.pdf.

Andersen, Ellen Ann. 2009. *Out of the Closets and into the Courts: Legal Opportunity Structure and Gay Rights Litigation*. Ann Arbor: University of Michigan Press.

Anderson, Lucas. 2009. "Kicking the National Habit: The Legal and Policy Arguments for Abolishing Private Prison Contracts." *Public Contract Law Journal*, 39 (1): 113–139.

Andrapalliyal, Vinita. 2013. "The CPS Took My Baby Away: Threats to Immigrant Parental Rights and a Proposed Federal Solution." *Harvard Law & Policy Review* 7: 173–197.

Antecol, Heather, and Kelly Bedard. 2006. "Unhealthy Assimilation: Why Do Immigrants Converge to American Health Status Levels?" *Demography* 43 (2): 337–360. https://link.springer.com/article/10.1353/dem.2006.0011.

Arcury, Thomas A., and Sara A. Quandt. 2007. "Delivery of Health Services to Migrant and Seasonal Farmworkers." *Annual Review of Public Health* 28 (1): 345–363.

Arsenault, Raymond. 2006. *Freedom Riders: 1961 and the Struggle for Racial Justice*. Oxford: Oxford University Press.

Asch, Steven, Barbara Leake, Ronald Anderson, and Lillian Gelberg. 1998. "Why Do Symptomatic Patients Delay Obtaining Care for Tuberculosis?" *American Journal of Respiratory and Critical Care Medicine* 157 (4): 1244–1248.

Associated Press. 2010. "Illegal Immigrants Leaving Arizona over New Law." CBS News. http://www.cbsnews.com/news/illegal-immigrants-leaving-arizona-over-new-law/.

Associated Press. 2016. "Arizona Sheriff Joe Arpaio is Officially Charged with Criminal Contempt in Racial Profiling Case." *Los Angeles Times*. http://www.latimes.com/nation/nationnow/la-na-arpaio-criminal-contempt-20161025-snap-story.html.

Barajas, R., N. Philipsen, and J. Brooks-Gunn. 2008. "Cognitive and Emotional Outcomes for Children in Poverty." In *Handbook of Families and Poverty*, edited by D. Crane and T. Heaton, 311–334. Thousand Oaks, CA: Sage Publications.

Barnett, Jessica C., and Marina S. Vornovitsky. 2016. *Health Insurance Coverage in the United States: 2015*. Washington, DC: U.S. Government Printing Office.

Baumeister, Lisa, and Norman Hearst. 1999. "Why Children's Health Is Threatened by Federal Immigration Policies." *Western Journal of Medicine* 171: 58–61.

Becker, Gay, Yewoubdar Beyene, and Pauline Ken. 2000. "Health, Welfare Reform, and Narratives of Uncertainty among Cambodian Refugees." *Culture, Medicine and Psychiatry* 24 (2): 139–163.

Beirich, Heidi, and Southern Poverty Law Center. 2011. "Georgia Governor Appoints Hate Group Leader to Immigration Board." September 2, 2011. http://www.splcenter.org/blog/2011/09/02/georgia-governor-appoints-nativist-hate-group-leader-to-immigration-board/.

Bell, Derrick A., Jr. 1995a. "Brown v. Board of Education and the Interest Convergence Dilemma." In *Critical Race Theory: The Key Writings That Formed the Movement*, edited by Kimberlé Crenshaw, Neil Gotanda, Gary Peller, and Kendall Thomas, 20–28. New York: New Press.

———. 1995b. "Serving Two Masters: Integration Ideals and Client Interests in School Desegregation Litigation." In *Critical Race Theory: The Key Writings That Formed the Movement*, edited by Kimberlé Crenshaw, Neil Gotanda, Gary Peller, and Kendall Thomas, 5–19. New York: New Press.

Berk, Marc L. 2001. "The Effect of Fear on Access to Care among Undocumented Latino Immigrants." *Journal of Immigrant Health* 3 (3): 151–156.

Berk, Marc L., Claudia L. Schur, Leo R. Chavez, and Martin Frankel. 2000. "Health Care Use among Undocumented Latino Immigrants: Is Free Health Care the Main Reason Why Latinos Come to the United States? A Unique Look at the Facts." *Health Affairs* 19 (4): 51–64.

Bess, Michael Kirkland, and Laura Shelton. 2008. *Across Imagined Boundaries: Understanding Mexican Migration to Georgia in a Transnational and Historical Context*. Statesboro: Georgia Southern University.

Biehl, João. *Will to live: AIDS therapies and the politics of survival*. Princeton, NJ: Princeton University Press, 2009.

Black Lives Matter. n.d. "About." Accessed July 19, 2018. https://blacklivesmatter.com/about/.

Blau, Max. 2013a. "How Grady Memorial Hospital Skirted Death." Creative Loafing Atlanta. http://clatl.com/atlanta/how-grady-memorial-hospital-skirted-death/Content?oid=7666302.

———. 2013b. "How Grady Memorial Hospital Skirted Death." Creative Loafing Atlanta. https://creativeloafing.com/content-170678-How-Grady-Memorial-Hospital-skirted-death.

———. 2013c. "This Georgia Hospital Shows Why Rejecting Medicaid Isn't Easy." *Washington Post*, June 26, 2013. http://www.washingtonpost.com/blogs/wonkblog/wp/2013/06/26/this-georgia-hospital-shows-why-rejecting-medicaid-isnt-easy/.

Blitzer, Jonathan. 2017. "An Underground College for Undocumented Immigrants." *New Yorker*, May 22, 2017. http://www.newyorker.com/magazine/2017/05/22/an-underground-college-for-undocumented-immigrants.

Boal, Augusto. 2000. *Theater of the Oppressed*. London: Pluto Press.

Boehm, Deborah. 2005. "The Safety Net of the Safety Net: How Federally Qualified Health Centers 'Subsidize' Medicaid Managed Care." *Medical Anthropology Quarterly* 19 (1): 47–63.

———. 2012. *Intimate Migrations: Gender, Family, and Illegality among Transnational Mexicans*. New York: New York University Press.

Bornstein, Robert F. 2006. "The Complex Relationship between Dependency and Domestic Violence: Converging Psychological Factors and Social Forces." *American Psychologist* 61 (6): 595–606.

Bostock, J.A.N., Maureen Plumpton, and Rebekah Pratt. 2009. "Domestic Violence against Women: Understanding Social Processes and Women's Experiences." *Journal of Community & Applied Social Psychology* 19 (2): 95–110.

Bourgois, Philippe I., and Jeffrey Schonberg. 2009. *Righteous Dopefiend*. Berkeley: University of California Press.

Branson-Potts, Hailey. 2017. "Before Stonewall, There Was the Black Cat; LGBTQ Leaders to Mark 50th Anniversary of Protests at Silver Lake Tavern." *Los Angeles Times*, February 8, 2017. http://www.latimes.com/local/lanow/la-me-ln-silver-lake-black-cat-lgbtq-20170208-story.html.

Braun, L. 2002. "Race, Ethnicity, and Health: Can Genetics Explain Disparities?" *Perspectives in Biology and Medicine* 45 (2): 159–174.

Brown, Anna, and Mark Hugo Lopez. 2013. *Mapping the Latino Population, by State, County and City*. Washington, DC: Pew Research Center.

Brown, Robbie. 2010. "Five Public Colleges in Georgia Ban Illegal-Immigrant Students." *New York Times*, October 13, 2010. http://www.nytimes.com/2010/10/14/us/14georgia.html?_r=0.

Browne, Irene, and Mary Odem. 2012. "'Juan Crow' in the Nuevo South?" *Du Bois Review: Social Science Research on Race* 9 (2): 321–337.

Bureau of Economic Analysis. 2016. "Gross Domestic Product by Metropolitan Area, 2015." https://www.bea.gov/news/2016/gross-domestic-product-metropolitan-area-2015.

Burress, Jim. 2012. "Georgia Immigration Law Trips Up Doctors and Nurses." National Public Radio, November 12, 2012. http://www.npr.org/blogs/health/2012/11/12/164950641/georgia-immigration-law-trips-up-doctors-and-nurses.

Calavita, Kitty. 1996. "The New Politics of Immigration: Balanced-Budget Conservatism and the Symbolism of Proposition 187." *Social Problems* 43: 284–305.

———. 2000. "The Paradoxes of Race, Class, Identity, and 'Passing': Enforcing the Chinese Exclusion Acts, 1882–1910." *Law & Social Inquiry* 25 (1): 1–40.

———. 2005. *Immigrants at the Margins: Law, Race, and Exclusion in Southern Europe*. Cambridge: Cambridge University Press.

Campbell, Kristina M. 2011. "The Road to SB 1070: How Arizona Became Ground Zero for the Immigrants' Rights Movement and the Continuing Struggle for Latino Civil Rights in America." *Harvard Latino Law Review* 14–21.

Capaldi, Deborah M., Naomi B. Knoble, Joann Wu Shortt, and Hyoun K. Kim. 2012. "A Systematic Review of Risk Factors for Intimate Partner Violence." *Partner Abuse* 3 (2): 231–280.

Capps, R., Marc R. Rosenblum, Muzaffar Christi, and Cristina Rodriguez. 2007. "Delegation and divergence: A Study of 287 (g) State and Local Immigration Enforcement." Washington, DC: Migration Policy Institute.

Carrasquero, Marian. 2018. "'I Can't Go without My Son,' a Mother Pleaded as She Was Deported to Guatemala." *New York Times*, June 17, 2018. https://www.nytimes.com/2018/06/17/us/immigration-deported-parents.html.

Carrion, I. V., H. Castañeda, D. Martinez-Tyson, and N. Kline. 2011. "Barriers Impeding Access to Primary Oral Health Care among Farmworker Families in Central Florida." *Social Work in Health Care* 50 (10): 828–844. https://doi.org/10.1080/00981389.2011.594491.

Cartwright, Elizabeth. 2011. "Immigrant Dreams: Legal Pathologies and Structural Vulnerabilities along the Immigration Continuum." *Medical Anthropology* 30 (5): 475–495.

Castañeda, Heide. 2010. "Im/Migration and Health: Conceptual, Methodological, and Theoretical Propositions for Applied Anthropology." *Napa Bulletin* 34 (1): 6–27.

———. 2012. "'Over-Foreignization,' or 'Unused Potential'? A Critical Review of Migrant Health in Germany and Responses toward Unauthorized Migration." *Social Science & Medicine* 74: 830–838.

———. 2019. *Borders of Belonging: Struggle and Solidarity in Mixed-status Immigrant Families.* Palo Alto, CA: Stanford University Press.

Castañeda, Heide, Iraida V. Carrion, Nolan Kline, and Dinorah Martinez Tyson. 2010. "False Hope: Effects of Social Class and Health Policy on Oral Health Inequalities for Migrant Farmworker Families." *Social Science and Medicine* 71 (11): 2028–2037. https://doi.org/10.1016/j.socscimed.2010.09.024.

Castañeda, Heide, Seth M. Holmes, Daniel S. Madrigal, Maria-Elena DeTrinidad Young, Naomi Beyeler, and James Quesada. 2015. "Immigration as a Social Determinant of Health." *Annual Review of Public Health* 36 (1): 1.1–1.18.

Castañeda, Heide, and Milena Melo. 2013. "Impact of the Affordable Care Act on Health Care Access for Mixed-Status Families." Annual Meeting of the American Anthropological Association. Chicago, IL, November 20–24.

———. 2014. "Health Care Access for Latino Mixed-Status Families: Barriers, Strategies, and Implications for Reform." *American Behavioral Scientist* 58 (14): 1891–1909.

Castro, Arachu, and Merrill Singer. 2004. *Unhealthy Health Policy: A Critical Anthropological Examination.* Lanham: Altamira Press.

Centers for Disease Control and Prevention. 2014. "National Chronic Kidney Disease Fact Sheet." http://www.cdc.gov/diabetes/pubs/factsheets/kidney.htm.

Chang, G. 2000. *Disposable Domestics: Immigrant Women Workers in the Global Economy.* Cambridge, MA: South End Press.

Chapman, Dan. 2014. "Metro Atlanta World's 44th Biggest Economy." *Atlanta Journal Constitution*, June 20, 2014. http://www.ajc.com/business/metro-atlanta-world-44th-biggest-economy/1dN3kdAzVC1hT4qj1LwrPM/.

Chaudry, Ajay, Randy Capps, Juan Manuel Pedroza, Rosa Maria Castaneda, Robert Santos, and Molly M. Scott. 2010. *Facing Our Future: Children in the Aftermath of Immigration Enforcement.* Washington, DC: The Urban Institute.

Chavez, Leo. 1997. "Immigration Reform and Nativism: The National Response to the Transnationalist Challenge." In *Immigrants Out!: The New Nativism and the Anti-immigrant Impulse in the United States*, edited by Juan F. Perea, 61–77. New York: New York University Press.

———. 2007. "The Condition of Illegality." *International Migration* 45 (3): 192–196.

———. 2013. *The Latino Threat: Constructing Immigrants, Citizens, and the Nation.* Stanford, CA: Stanford University Press.

Chavez, Nicole. 2018. "Justice Department Won't Defend DACA in Texas Lawsuit." CNN, June 9, 2018. https://www.cnn.com/2018/06/09/politics/daca-lawsuit-texas/index.html.

Clark, Brietta R. 2008. "The Immigrant Health Care Narrative and What It Tells Us about the US Health Care System." *Annals of Health Law* 17: 229–278.

Cleaveland, Carol, and Emily S. Ihara. 2012. "'They Treat Us Like Pests': Undocumented Immigrant Experiences Obtaining Health Care in the Wake of a 'Crackdown' Ordinance." *Journal of Human Behavior in the Social Environment* 22 (7): 771–788.

Cobb County Sheriff's Office. 2015. "Sheriff Neil Warren." http://www.cobbsheriff.org/sheriff -neil-warren/.

Coleman, Mathew. 2007. "Immigration Geopolitics beyond the Mexico-US Border." *Antipode* 39 (1): 54–76.

Colino, Stacey. 1995. "The Fallout from Proposition 197." *Human Rights* 22 (1): 16–17.

Conyers, John. 2007. "The 2005 Reauthorization of the Violence Against Women Act Why Congress Acted to Expand Protections to Immigrant Victims." *Violence against Women* 13 (5): 457–468.

Coughlin, Teresa A., and David Liska. 1997. "The Medicaid Disproportionate Share Hospital Payment Program: Background and Issues." The Urban Institute. https://www.urban.org /sites/default/files/publication/71236/307025-The-Medicaid-Disproportionate-Share -Hospital-Payment-Program.PDF.

Crawford, Tom. 2013. "Nursing Licenses Held Up by Immigration Law." February 5, 2013. http://gareport.com/story/2013/02/05/nursing-licenses-held-up-by-immigration-law/.

Crenshaw, Kimberlé. 1989. "Demarginalizing the Intersection of Race and Sex: A Black Feminist Critique of Antidiscrimination Doctrine, Feminist Theory and Antiracist Politics." *University of Chicago Legal Forum*, 1: 139–167.

———. 1995. "Mapping the Margins: Intersectionality, Identity, Politics, and Violence against Women of Color." In *Critical Race Theory: The Key Writings That Formed the Movement*, edited by Kimberlé Crenshaw, 357–383. New York: New Press.

Davis, Karyl Alice. 2004. "Unlocking the Door by Giving Her the Key: A Comment on the Adequacy of the U-Visa as a Remedy." *Alabama Law Review* 56: 557–575.

De Genova, Nicholas. 2002. "Migrant 'Illegality' and Deportability in Everyday Life." *Annual Review of Anthropology*, 31 (1): 419–447.

———. 2004. "The Legal Production of Mexican/Migrant 'Illegality.'" *Latino Studies* 2 (2): 160–185.

———. 2005. *Working the Boundaries: Race, Space, and "Illegality" in Mexican Chicago*. Durham, NC: Duke University Press.

De León, Jason. 2015. *The Land of Open Graves: Living and Dying on the Migrant Trail*. Vol. 36. Oakland: University of California Press.

Delgado, Richard. 1995. "The Imperial Scholar: Reflections on a Review of Civil Rights Literature." In *Critical Race Theory: The Key Writings That Formed the Movement*, edited by Kimberlé Crenshaw, Neil Gotanda, Gary Peller, and Kendall Thomas, 46–57. New York: New Press.

Delgado, Richard, and Jean Stefancic. 2012. *Critical Race Theory: An Introduction*. 2nd ed. New York: New York University Press.

Department of Homeland Security. 2018. "Fact Sheet: Zero Tolerance Immigration Prosecutions—Families." June 15, 2018. https://www.dhs.gov/news/2018/06/15/fact-sheet -zero-tolerance-immigration-prosecutions-families.

Detention Watch Network. n.d. "Immigration Detention 101." https://www.detention watchnetwork.org/issues/detention-101. Accessed January 25, 2019.

Dewan, Shaila, and Kevin Sack. 2008. "A Safety-Net Hospital Falls Into Financial Crisis." *New York Times*, January 8, 2008. http://www.nytimes.com/2008/01/08/us/08grady.html ?pagewanted=all&_r=0.

Dinnerstein, Leonard. 2008. *The Leo Frank Case*. Athens: University of Georgia Press.

Dreby, Joanna. 2012a. "The Burden of Deportation on Children in Mexican Immigrant Families." *Journal of Marriage and Family* 74 (4): 829–845.

————. 2012b. *How Today's Immigration Enforcement Policies Impact Children, Families, and Communities: A View from the Ground.* Washington, DC: Center for American Progress. http://www.americanprogress.org/wp-content/uploads/2012/08DrebyImmigration FamiliesFINAL.pdf.

El Refugio. 2018. No title. https://www.elrefugiostewart.org/el-refugio-receives-gift-from-full -frontal-with-samantha-bee/. December 18.

Ellsberg, Mary, Henrica A. F. M. Jansen, Lori Heise, Charlotte H. Watts, and Claudia Garcia-Moreno. 2008. "Intimate Partner Violence and Women's Physical and Mental Health in the WHO Multi-country Study on Women's Health and Domestic Violence: An Observational Study." *The Lancet* 371 (9619): 1165–1172.

Ellwood, Marilyn R., and Leighton Ku. 1998. "Welfare and Immigration Reforms: Unintended Side Effects for Medicaid." *Health Affairs* 17 (3): 137–151.

Emporis. 2019a. "Cities with the Most Skyscrapers." https://www.emporis.com/statistics/most -skyscraper-cities-worldwide.

Emporis. 2019b. "U.S.A.'s Tallest Buildings-Top 25." https://www.emporis.com/statistics/tallest -buildings/country/100185/usa.

Erez, Edna, Madelaine Adelman, and Carol Gregory. 2008. "Intersections of Immigration and Domestic Violence: Voices of Battered Immigrant Women." *Feminist Criminology* 4 (1): 32–56.

Escobar, Javier I., Hoyos Nervi Constanza, and Michael A. Gara. 2009. "Immigration and Mental Health: Mexican Americans in the United States." *Harvard Review of Psychiatry* 8 (2): 64–72.

Faigin, David, and Catherine Stein. 2010. "The Power of Theater to Promote Individual Recovery and Social Change." *Psychiatric Services* 61 (3): 306–308.

Fairchild, Amy L. 2004. "Policies of Inclusion: Immigrants, Disease, Dependency, and American Immigration Policy at the Dawn and Dusk of the 20th Century." *American Journal of Public Health* 94 (4): 528–539.

Feagin, Joe R. 1997. "Old Poison in New Bottles: The Deep Roots of Modern Nativism." In *Immigration Reform and Nativism: The Nationalist Response to the Transnationalist Challenge*, edited by Juan F. Perea, 13–43. New York: New York University Press.

Feldman, Allen. 1991. *Formations of Violence: The Narrative of the Body and Political Terror in Northern Ireland.* Chicago: University of Chicago Press.

————. 1997a. "Retaliate and Punish: Political Violence as Form and Memory in Northern Ireland." *Eire-Ireland* 33 (1): 195–235.

————. (1997b). "Violence and Vision: the Prosthetics and Aesthetics of Terror." *Public Culture* 10 (1): 24–60.

Fernandez, Manny. 2018. "Inside the Former Walmart That Is Now a Shelter for Almost 1,500 Migrant Children." *New York Times*, June 14, 2018. https://www.nytimes.com/2018/06/14 /us/family-separation-migrant-children-detention.html.

Finneran, Catherine, and Rob Stephenson. 2013. "Gay and Bisexual Men's Perceptions of Police Helpfulness in Response to Male-Male Intimate Partner Violence." *Western Journal of Emergency Medicine* 14 (4): 354–362.

Foley, Elise. 2014. "Georgia Republicans Aim to Keep Driver's Licenses from Dreamers." *Huffington Post*, February 24, 2014. http://www.huffingtonpost.com/2014/02/24/georgia -republicans-dreamers_n_4849149.html.

Foucault, Michel. 1978. *The History of Sexuality. Volume I: An Introduction.* New York: Vintage.

————. 1980. *Power/knowledge: Selected Interviews and Other Writings, 1972–1977.* New York: Pantheon.

————. 2003. *Society Must Be Defended: Lectures at the Collége de France, 1975–76.* New York: Picador USA.

Fragomen, Austin T. 1997. "The Illegal Immigration Reform and Immigrant Responsibility Act of 1996: An Overview." *International Migration Review* 31 (2): 438–460.

Frank, Richard G., Thomas G. McGuire, and Joseph P. Newhouse. 1995. "Risk Contracts in Managed Mental Health Care." *Health Affairs* 14 (3): 50–64.

Freeman, Alan David. 1995. "Legitimizing Racial Discrimination through Antidiscrimination Law: A Critical Review of Supreme Court Doctrine." In *Critical Race Theory: The Key Writings That Formed the Movement*, edited by Kimberlé Crenshaw, Neil Gotanda, Gary Peller, and Kendall Thomas, 29–45. New York: New Press.

Friends of Stacey Y. Abrams. 2014. "Stacey's Story." http://staceyabrams.com/about/bio/.

Fujiwara, Lynn H. 2005. "Immigrant Rights Are Human Rights: The Reframing of Immigrant Entitlement and Welfare." *Social Problems* 52 (1): 79–101.

Gamble, Molly. 2013a. "50 Largest Public Hospitals in America." Becker's Hospital Review. http://www.beckershospitalreview.com/lists-and-statistics/50-largest-public-hospitals -in-america-2013.html.

———. 2013b. "Safety-Nets: Can They Go from 'Last Resort' to 'Hospitals of Choice'?" Becker's Hospital Review. http://www.beckershospitalreview.com/hospital-management -administration/safety-nets-can-they-go-from-last-resort-to-hospitals-of-choice.html.

García, Angela S. 2013. "Return to Sender? A Comparative Analysis of Immigrant Communities in 'Attrition through Enforcement' Destinations." *Ethnic and Racial Studies* 36 (11): 1849–1870.

Garfield, Rachel, and Anthony Damico. 2016. "The Coverage Gap: Uninsured Poor Adults in States That Do Not Expand Medicaid—an Update." Kaiser Commission on Medicaid and the Uninsured. http://kff.org/health-reform/issue-brief/the-coverage-gap-uninsured-poor -adults-in-states-that-do-not-expand-medicaid-an-update/.

Gebisa, Ebba. "Constitutional Concerns with the Enforcement and Expansion of Expedited Removal." *University of Chicago Legal Forum*. 1 (18) 565–589.

Georgia Department of Agriculture. 2012. "Report on Agriculture Labor." http://agr.georgia .gov/AgLaborReport.pdf.

Georgia January 20th Coalition. n.d. "About." https://gaj20.wordpress.com/about/. Accessed January 23, 2019.

Georgia Latino Alliance for Human Rights. 2014. "DeKalb County Sheriff Rejects ICE Requests." December 16, 2014. http://www.glahr.org/our-work/latest-news/item/53-dekalb -county-sheriff-rejects-unconstitutional-detention-ice.

Georgia Restaurant Association. n.d. "Join Us in Opposing Costly Immigration Bills (HB-87/ SB-40)." http://www.garestaurants.org/resources/Documents/immigration.pdf. Accessed December 10, 2015.

Georgia State Office of Rural Health. n.d. "Georgia's Rural Counties." https://dch.georgia.gov /sites/dch.georgia.gov/files/imported/vgn/images/portal/cit_1210/19/60/127722716 GeorgiaRuralcounties.pdf. Accessed January 24, 2019.

Gladstone, Rick, and Satoshi Sugiyama. July 1, 2018. "Trump's Travel Ban: How It Works and Who Is Affected." *The New York Times*. https://www.nytimes.com/2018/07/01/world /americas/travel-ban-trump-how-it-works.html.

Goffman, Erving. 1986. Frame Analysis. *An Essay on the Organization of Experience*. Boston: Northeastern University Press.

Goldade, Kathryn. 2009. "'Health Is Hard Here' or 'Health for All'?" *Medical Anthropology Quarterly* 23 (4): 483–503.

Gomberg-Muñoz, Ruth. 2016. *Becoming Legal: Immigration Law and Mixed Status Families*. New York: Oxford University Press.

Gordon, Edmund T. 1991. "Anthropology and Liberation." In *Decolonizing Anthropology*, edited by Faye V. Harrison, 149–167. Washington, DC: American Anthropological Association.

Gordon, Ian, and Tasneem Raja. 2012. "164 Anti-immigration Laws Passed Since 2010? A MoJo Analysis." *Mother Jones*, March/April 2012. http://motherjones.com/politics/2012/03/anti -immigration-law-database.

Gostin, Lawrence O. 2010. *Public Health Law & Ethics: A Reader.* 2nd ed. Berkeley: University of California Press.

———. 2008. *Public Health Law: Power, Duty, Restraint.* 2nd ed. Berkeley and Los Angeles: University of California Press.

Grady Health System. c2019. "Billing and Insurance." http://www.gradyhealth.org/billing-and -insurance. Accessed January 22, 2019.

———. c2018. "Grady EMS Paramedic Training." http://grady-ems.org/paramedic/. Accessed January 22, 2019.

Gravlee, Clarence C. 2009. "How Race Becomes Biology: Embodiment of Social Inequality." *American Journal of Physical Anthropology* 139 (1): 47–57. http://onlinelibrary.wiley.com/doi /10.100.

Green, Linda. 1994. "Fear as a Way of Life." *Cultural Anthropology* 9 (2): 227–256.

———. 1999. *Fear as a Way of Life: Mayan Windows in Rural Guatemala.* New York: Columbia University Press.

Greenwood, Gregory L., Michael V. Relf, Bu Huang, Lance M. Pollack, Jesse A. Canchola, and Joseph A. Catania. 2002. "Battering Victimization among a Probability-Based Sample of Men Who Have Sex with Men." *American Journal of Public Health* 92 (12): 1964–1969.

Grillo, Jery. 2010. "The Immigration Dilemma." *Georgia Trend.* http://www.georgiatrend.com /December-2010/The-Immigration-Dilemma/.

Gusterson, H. 1997. "Studying Up Revisited." *PoLAR: Political and Legal Anthropology Review* 20 (1): 114–119.

Hagan, Jacqueline, Nestor Rodriguez, Randy Capps, and Nika Kabiri. 2003. "The Effects of Recent Welfare and Immigration Reforms on Immigrants' Access to Health Care." *International Migration Review* 37 (2): 444–463.

Hale, Charles R. 2008. "Introduction." In *Engaging Contradictions: Theory, Politics and Methods of Activist Scholarship*, 1–28. Berkeley: University of California Press.

Hardy, Lisa J., Christina M. Getrich, Julio C. Quezada, Amanda Guay, Raymond J. Michalowski, and Eric Henley. 2012. "A Call for Further Research on the Impact of State-Level Immigration Policies on Public Health." *American Journal of Public Health* 102 (7): 1250–1253.

Harvey, David. 2007. *A Brief History of Neoliberalism.* New York: Oxford University Press.

Health Students Taking Action Together. 2016. "Our History." http://www.hstatga.org/our -history/.

Heidbrink, Lauren. 2014. *Migrant Youth, Transnational Families, and the State: Care and Contested Interests.* Philadelphia: University of Pennsylvania Press.

Hertzman, Clyde, and Tom Boyce. 2010. "How Experience Gets Under the Skin to Create Gradients in Developmental Health." *Annual Review of Public Health* 31: 329–347.

Heyman, J.M.C. 2008. "Constructing a Virtual Wall: Race and Citizenship in US-Mexico Border Policing." *Journal of the Southwest*, 50 (3): 305–333.

———. 2009. "'You Lie!': Going Beyond the Obama-Wilson Debate." Access Denied: A Conversation on Im/migration and Health. http://accessdeniedblog.wordpress.com/2009 /12/01/you-lie-going-beyond-the-obama-wilson-debate/.

Heyman, J.M.C., G. G. Núñez, and V. Talavera. 2009. "Healthcare Access and Barriers for Unauthorized Immigrants in El Paso County, Texas." *Family & Community Health* 32 (1): 4–21.

Hiemstra, N. 2010. "Immigrant 'Illegality' as Neoliberal Governmentality in Leadville, Colorado." *Antipode* 42 (1): 74–102.

Himmelgreen, David, Nancy Romero Daza, Elizabeth Cooper, and Dinorah Martinez. 2007. "'I Don't Make the Soups Anymore': Pre- to Post-Migration Dietary and Lifestyle Changes among Latinos Living in West-Central Florida." *Ecology of Food and Nutrition* 46 (5): 427–444.

Hoffman, Beatrix. 2006. "Sympathy and Exclusion: Access to Health Care for Undocumented Immigrants in the United States." In *A Death Retold: Jesica Santillan, the Bungled Transplant, and Paradoxes in Medical Citizenship,* edited by K. Wailoo, J. Livingston, and P. J. Guarnaccia. Chapel Hill: University of North Carolina Press.

Holmes, Seth. 2013. *Fresh Fruit, Broken Bodies: Migrant Farmworkers in the United States.* Berkeley: University of California Press.

Hondagneu-Sotelo, Pierrette. 2001. *Domestica: Immigrant Workers and Their Employers.* Berkeley: University of California Press. Google Scholar.

Horton, Sarah Bronwen. 2004. "Different Subjects: The Health Care System's Participation in the Differential Construction of the Cultural Citizenship of Cuban Refugees and Mexican Immigrants." *Medical Anthropology Quarterly* 18 (4): 472–489.

———. 2009. "A Mother's Heart Is Weighed Down with Stones: A Phenomenological Approach to the Experience of Transnational Motherhood." *Culture, Medicine, and Psychiatry* 33 (1): 21–40.

———. 2014. "Debating 'Medical Citizenship': Policies Shaping Undocumented Immigrants' Learned Avoidance of the U.S. Health Care System." In *Hidden Lives and Human Rights in the United States: Understanding the Controversies and Tragedies of Undocumented Immigration,* edited by Lois Ann Lorentzen. Vol. 2, 297–320. Santa Barbara, CA: Praeger.

———. 2016a. "From 'Deportability' to 'Denounce-Ability': New Forms of Labor Subordination in an Era of Governing Immigration through Crime." *PoLAR: Political and Legal Anthropology Review* 39 (2): 312–326. https://doi.org/10.1111/plar.12196.

———. 2016b. *They Leave Their Kidneys in the Fields: Illness, Injury, and Illegality among US Farmworkers.* Vol. 40. Oakland: University of California Press.

Horton, Sarah B., and Judith C. Barker. 2010a. "A Latino Oral Health Paradox? Using Ethnography to Specify the Biocultural Factors behind Epidemiological Models." *Napa Bulletin* 34 (1): 68–83. https://doi.org/10.1111/j.1556-4797.2010.01052.x.

———. 2010b. "Stigmatized Biologies: Examining Oral Health Disparities for Mexican American Farmworker Children and Their Cumulative Effects." *Medical Anthropology Quarterly* 24 (2): 199–219.

Howard, Leigh Anne. 2004. "Speaking Theatre/Doing Pedagogy: Re-visiting Theatre of the Oppressed." *Communication Education* 53 (3): 217–233.

Hsia, Renee Y., Arthur L. Kellermann, and Yu-Chu Shen. 2011. "Factors Associated with Closures of Emergency Departments in the United States." *Journal of the American Medical Association* 305 (19): 1978–1985.

Hsieh, Hui-Min, and Gloria J. Bazzoli. 2012. "Medicaid Disproportionate Share Hospital Payment: How Does It Impact Hospitals' Provision of Uncompensated Care?" *INQUIRY: The Journal of Health Care Organization, Provision, and Financing* 49 (3): 254–267.

Huang, Priscilla. 2008. "Anchor Babies, Over-Breeders, and the Population Bomb: The Reemergence of Nativism and Population Control in Anti-immigration Policies." *Harvard Law & Policy Review* 2: 385–406.

Huang, Z. J., M. Y. Stella, and R. Ledsky. 2006. "Health Status and Health Service Access and Use among Children in US Immigrant Families." *American Journal of Public Health* 96 (4): 634–640.

Human Impact Partners. 2013. *Family Unity, Family Health: How Family-Focused Immigration Reform Will Mean Better Health for Children and Families.* Oakland, CA: Human Impact Partners.

Hyatt, Susan Brinn. 2001. "From Citizen to Volunteer: Neoliberal Governance and the Erasure of Poverty." In *The New Poverty Studies: The Ethnography of Power, Politics, and Impoverished People in the United States*, edited by Judith Goode and Jeff Maskovsky, 201–235. New York: New York University Press.

Ibarra, Ana B., and Chad Terhune. 2017. "California Withdraws Bid to Allow Undocumented to Buy Unsubsidized Plans." January 20, 2017. http://khn.org/news/california-withdraws -bid-to-allow-undocumented-immigrants-to-buy-unsubsidized-obamacare-plans/.

Immigration and Customs Enforcement. July 12, 2018. "ICE Detainee Passes Away at Georgia Hospital." https://www.ice.gov/news/releases/ice-detainee-passes-away-georgia-hospital-1.

Immigration Policy Center. August 13, 2013. "An Immigration Stimulus: The Economic Benefits of a Legalization Program." https://www.americanimmigrationcouncil.org/research /immigration-stimulus-economic-benefits-legalization-program.

Indivisible Project. 2019. "Introduction to the Guide." https://indivisible.org/guide.

Inda, Jonathan Xavier, and Julie A. Dowling. 2013. "Introduction: Governing Migrant Illegality." In *Governing Immigration through Crime: A Reader*, edited by Jonathan Xavier Inda and Julie A. Dowling, 1–36. Stanford, CA: Stanford University Press.

Isin, E. F., and B. S. Turner. 2002. *Handbook of Citizenship Studies*. London: Sage Publications.

Johnson, Jeh Charles. 2014. "Memorandum: Secure Communities." Edited by Thomas S. Winkowski, Megan Mack, and Philip A. McNamara. http://www.dhs.gov/sites/default /files/publications/14_1120_memo_secure_communities.pdf.

Johnson, Kevin R. 2009. "The Intersection of Race and Class in US Immigration Law and Enforcement." *Law and Contemporary Problems* 72: 1.

Jordain Carney. 2017. "Sanders: Trump's revised travel ban 'racist and anti-Islamic.'" The Hill. https://thehill.com/blogs/floor-action/senate/322521-sanders-trumps-revised-ban -racist-and-anti-islamic.

Jordan, Jan. 2004. "Beyond Belief? Police, Rape and Women's Credibility." *Criminal Justice* 4 (1): 29–59.

Kaiser Commission on Facts. 2006. "Medicaid and SCHIP Eligibility for Immigrants." Henry J. Kaiser Family Foundation. http://www.kff.org/medicaid/upload/7492.pdf.

———. 2008. "Summary: Five Basic Facts on Immigrants and Their Health Care." Henry J. Kaiser Family Foundation. http://www.kff.org/medicaid/upload/7761.pdf.

Kaiser Family Foundation. 2015. "Total Number of Medicare Beneficiaries." http://www.kff.org /medicare/state-indicator/total-medicare-beneficiaries/?currentTimeframe=0&sort Model=%7B%22colId%22:%22Location%22,%22sort%22:%22asc%22%7D.

Karkaria, Urvaksh. 2008. "Woodruff Bails Out Grady Hospital with $200M in Aid." *Atlanta Business Chronicle*, April 7, 2008. http://www.bizjournals.com/atlanta/stories/2008/04/07 /daily14.html.

Kenney, Genevieve M., and Michael Huntress. 2012. *The Affordable Care Act: Coverage Implications and Issues for Immigrant Families*. Washington, DC: US Department of Health and Human Services.

Khalid, Asma. 2016. "Latinos Will Never Vote for a Republican, and Other Myths about Hispanics from 2016." National Public Radio, December 22, 2016. http://www.npr.org/2016 /12/22/506347254/latinos-will-never-vote-for-a-republican-and-other-myths-about -hispanics-from-20.

Kimport, Katrina. 2017. "More Than a Physical Burden: Women's Mental and Emotional Work in Preventing Pregnancy." *Journal of Sex Research* 55 (9): 1096–1105.

Kline, Nolan. 2010. "Disparate Power and Disparate Resources: Collaboration between Faith-Based and Activist Organizations for Central Florida Farmworkers." *Napa Bulletin* 33 (8): 126–142.

———. 2012. "There's Nowhere I Can Go to Get Help, and I Have Tooth Pain Right Now": The Oral Health Syndemic among Migrant Farmworkers in Florida." *Annals of Anthropological Practice.* Vol. 36. https://doi.org/10.1111/napa.12010.

———. 2017. "Pathogenic Policy: Immigrant Policing, Fear, and Parallel Medical Systems in the US South." *Medical Anthropology: Cross Cultural Studies in Health and Illness* 36 (4): 396–410. https://doi.org/10.1080/01459740.2016.1259621.

———. 2018a. "It's Too Risky to Leave the House:" Immigrant Policing and Health-Related Mobility. In *Healthcare in Motion: Mobilities in Health Service Delivery and Access,* edited by Cecilia Vindrola, Anne Pfister, and Ginger Johnson. New York and Oxford: Berghahn Books.

———. 2018b. "'How Will I Get My Skull Back?' The Embodied Consequences of Immigrant Policing." In *Forced Out, Fenced In: Immigration Tales from the Field,* edited by Tanya Golash-Boza. New York: Oxford University Press.

———. 2018c. "Life, Death, and Dialysis: Medical Repatriation and Liminal Life among Undocumented Kidney Failure Patients in the United States." *PoLAR: Political and Legal Anthropology Review* 41 (2): 216–230.

Kobach, Kris W. 2008. "Attrition through Enforcement: A Rational Approach to Illegal Immigration." *Tulane Journal of International and Comparative Law* 15: 155–163.

Kopan, Tal. 2018. "Trump Admin Thought Family Separations Would Deter Immigrants. They Haven't." CNN, June 18, 2018. https://www.cnn.com/2018/06/18/politics/family -separation-deterrence-dhs/index.html.

Kretsedemas, Philip, and David C. Brotherton. 2004. "Open Markets, Militarized Borders? Immigration Enforcement Today." In *Keeping Out the Other: A Critical Introduction to Immigration Enforcement Today,* edited by David C. Brotherton and Philip Kretsedemas, 1–28. New York: Columbia University Press.

Ku, Leighton., and Sheetal Matani. 2001. "Left Out: Immigrants' Access to Health Care and Insurance." *Health Affairs* 20 (1): 247–256.

Ku, Leighton, and Fouad Pervez. 2010. "Documenting citizenship in Medicaid: The struggle between ideology and evidence." *Journal of Health Politics, Policy and Law* 35 (1): 5–28.

Kuck, Charles. 2011. "The Georgia Immigration Enforcement Review Board." *Musings on Immigration* (blog). September 6, 2011. http://musingsonimmigration.blogspot.com/2011/09 /georgia-immigration-enforcement-review.html.

Kullgren, J. T. 2003. "Restrictions on Undocumented Immigrants' Access to Health Services: The Public Health Implications of Welfare Reform." *American Journal of Public Health* 93 (10): 1630–1633.

Lacey, Marc, and Salvador Rodriguez. 2011. "Arizona Sues Federal Government for Failing to Enforce Immigration." *New York Times,* February 10, 2011. http://thecaucus.blogs.nytimes .com/2011/02/10/arizona-plans-to-sue-federal-government/?_r=o.

LaRocco, Susan. 2011. "Treatment Options for Patients with Kidney Failure." *AJN American Journal of Nursing* 111 (10): 57–62.

LeBrón, Alana M. W., William D. Lopez, Keta Cowan, Nicole L. Novak, Olivia Temrowski, Maria Ibarra-Frayre, and Jorge Delva. 2018. "Restrictive ID Policies: Implications for Health Equity." *Journal of Immigrant and Minority Health* 20 (2): 255–260.

Lee, Tiana Mayere. 2004. "An EMTALA Primer: The Impact of Changes in the Emergency Medicine Landscape on EMTALA Compliance and Enforcement." *Annals of Health Law* 13 (1): 145–178.

Leerkes, Arjen, Mark Leach, and James Bachmeier. 2012. "Borders behind the Border: An Exploration of State-Level Differences in Migration Control and Their Effects on US Migration Patterns." *Journal of Ethnic and Migration Studies* 38 (1): 111–129.

Lende, D. H., and A. Lachiondo. 2009. "Embodiment and Breast Cancer among African American Women." *Qualitative Health Research* 19 (2): 216–228.

Leventhal, T., and J. Brooks-Gunn. 2004. "Diversity in Developmental Trajectories across Adolescence: Neighborhood Influences." In *Handbook of Adolescent Psychology*, 2nd ed., edited by R. Lerner and L. Steinberg, 451–486. Hoboken, NJ: John Wiley & Sons.

Linehan, Kathryn. 2013. "CMS's Proposed Rule Implementing the ACA-Mandated Medicaid DSH Reductions." *National Health Policy Forum, George Washington University* 849: 1–11.

Linthicum, Kate. 2014. "Obama Ends Secure Communities Program as Part of Immigration Action." *Los Angeles Times*, November 21, 2014. http://www.latimes.com/local/california/la-me-1121-immigration-justice-20141121-story.html.

Livingston, Gretchen. 2009. "Pew Research Center: Hispanics, Health Insurance and Health Care Access." September 25, 2009. http://www.pewhispanic.org/2009/09/25/hispanics-health-insurance-and-health-care-access/.

Lock, Margaret, and Vinh-Kim Nguyen. 2010. *An Anthropology of Biomedicine*. Malden, MA: Wiley-Blackwell.

Lohr, Kathy. 2012. "Georgia Town Ranks as City with Worst U.S. Job Loss." NPR, August 10, 2012. http://www.npr.org/2012/08/10/158556689/georgia-town-ranks-as-city-with-worst-u-s-job-loss.

Lopes, Harrison, and Adam Thomas. 2014. "The Relationships between Permissive and Restrictive State Immigration Laws and Violent Crime Rates in Big Cities." Master's Degree Thesis, Georgetown University.

Lopez, William D., Daniel J. Kruger, Jorge Delva, Mikel Llanes, Charo Ledón, Adreanne Waller, Melanie Harner, Ramiro Martinez, Laura Sanders, and Margaret Harner. 2016. "Health Implications of an Immigration Raid: Findings from a Latino Community in the Midwestern United States." *Journal of Immigrant and Minority Health*, 19 (3): 702–708

Lopez, William D., Nicole L. Novak, Melanie Harner, Ramiro Martinez, and Julia S. Seng. 2018. "The Traumatogenic Potential of Law Enforcement Home Raids: An Exploratory Report." *Traumatology* 24 (3): 193–199.

Lutz, Catherine. 2014. "The US Car Colossus and the Production of Inequality." *American Ethnologist* 41 (2): 232–245.

Madara, James L. 2018. "AMA Urges Administration to Withdraw 'Zero Tolerance' Policy." American Medical Association, June 20, 2018. https://www.ama-assn.org/ama-urges-administration-withdraw-zero-tolerance-policy.

Manderson, Lenore, and Carolyn Smith-Morris. 2010. "Introduction." In *Chronic Conditions, Fluid States: Chronicity and the Anthropology of Illness*, edited by Lenore Manderson and Carolyn Smith-Morris, 1–20. New Brunswick, NJ: Rutgers University Press.

Marcus, George E. "Ethnography in/of the world system: The emergence of multi-sited ethnography." *Annual review of Anthropology* 24 (1): 95–117.

Marietta Daily Journal. 2018. "AROUND TOWN: Cobb Sheriff to Congress: Stand up to ICE Criticism; GOP Float Flap" July 6, 2018. https://www.mdjonline.com/opinion/around-town-cobb-sheriff-to-congress-stand-up-to-ice/article_f25c3afe-816b-11e8-8f0e-439918b7707a.html.

Markel, Howard, and Alexandra Minna Stern. 1999. "Which face? Whose nation? Immigration, public health, and the construction of disease at America's ports and borders, 1891–1928." *American Behavioral Scientist* 42 (9): 1314–1331.

Marrow, Hellen B. 2012. "Deserving to a Point: Unauthorized Immigrants in San Francisco's Universal Access Healthcare Model." *Social Science & Medicine* 74 (6): 846–854.

Maskovsky, Jeff. 2000. "Managing the Poor: Neoliberalism, Medicaid HMOs and the Triumph of Consumerism among the Poor." *Medical Anthropology* 19 (2): 121–146.

———. 2005. "Do People Fail Drugs, or Do Drugs Fail People? The Discourse of Adherence." *Transforming Anthropology* 13 (2): 136–142.

Massey, Douglas S., and Karen A. Pren. 2012. "Unintended Consequences of US Immigration Policy: Explaining the Post-1965 Surge from Latin America." *Population and Development Review* 38 (1): 1–29.

Mbembe, Achille, and Libby Meintjes. 2003. "Necropolitics." *Public Culture* 15 (1): 11–40.

McDonald, R. Robin. 2014. "Hospital, Medical Firm CEOs to Plead Guilty to Kickbacks." *Daily Report.* http://www.dailyreportonline.com/id=1202665296890/Hospital-Medical-Firm -CEOs-to-Plead-Guilty-to-Kickbacks#ixzz3OwpXYwZg.

McEwen, Bruce S. 2004. "Protection and Damage from Acute and Chronic Stress: Allostasis and Allostatic Overload." *Annals of the New York Academy of Sciences* 1032: 1–7.

———. 2012. "Brain on Stress: How the Social Environment Gets Under the Skin." *Proceedings of the National Academy of Sciences* 109 (Supplement 2): 17180–17185.

McLeroy, Kenneth R., Daniel Bibeau, Allan Steckler, and Karen Glanz. 1988. "An Ecological Perspective on Health Promotion Programs." *Health Education & Behavior* 15 (4): 351–377.

Mechanic, Robert. 2004. "Medicaid's Disproportionate Share Hospital Program: Complex Structure, Critical Payments." *National Health Policy Forum, George Washington University.* 1–24. http://www.nhpf.org/library/background-papers/BP_MedicaidDSH_09-14-04.pdf.

Medina, Jennifer. 2016. "California Moves to Allow Undocumented Immigrants to Buy Insurance." *New York Times,* September 15, 2016. https://www.nytimes.com/2016/09/16/us /california-moves-to-allow-undocumented-immigrants-to-buy-insurance.html.

Menjívar, Cecilia. 2014. "The 'Poli-Migra': Multilayered Legislation, Enforcement Practices, and What We Can Learn about and from Today's Approaches." *American Behavioral Scientist,* 58 (13): 1805–1819.

Menjívar, Cecilia, and Olivia Salcido. 2002. "Immigrant Women and Domestic Violence: Common Experiences in Different Countries." *Gender & Society* 16 (6): 898–920.

Migration Policy Institute. 2014. "Current and Historical Numbers and Shares: How Many Immigrants Reside in the United States?" http://www.migrationpolicy.org/article /frequently-requested-statistics-immigrants-and-immigration-united-states#1.

Miklavcic, Alessandra. 2011. "Canada's Non-status Immigrants: Negotiating Access to Health Care and Citizenship." *Medical Anthropology* 30 (5): 496–517. https://doi.org/10.1080 /01459740.2011.579586.

Miller, Andy. 2011a. "Dialysis Deal Runs Out, Leaving 22 in Limbo." Georgia Health News, September 1, 2011. http://www.georgiahealthnews.com/2011/09/dialysis-deal-runs-out-leaving -22-limbo/.

———. 2011b. "Grady, Fresenius Reach Deal on Dialysis." Georgia Health News, September 7, 2011. http://www.georgiahealthnews.com/2011/09/grady-fresenius-reach-deal -patients-dialysis/.

———. 2017. "Georgia Has Too Few Nurses, and the Problem Could Get Much Worse." Georgia Health News, January 17, 2017. http://www.georgiahealthnews.com/2017/01 /georgia-nurses-problem-worse/.

Miller, Jim. 2017. "Fearing Trump, California Drops Undocumented Health Insurance Request." *Sacramento Bee,* January 18, 2017. http://www.sacbee.com/news/politics-government /capitol-alert/article127360849.html.

Miller, T. A. 2005. "Blurring the Boundaries between Immigration and Crime Control after September 11th." *Boston College Third World Law Journal* 25 (1): 1–43.

Mishtal, Joanna Z. 2009. "Matters of 'Conscience': The Politics of Reproductive Healthcare in Poland." *Medical Anthropology Quarterly* 23 (2): 161–183.

Mixon, Gregory. 1997. "'Good Negro—Bad Negro': The Dynamics of Race and Class in Atlanta during the Era of the 1906 Riot." *Georgia Historical Quarterly* 81 (3): 593–621.

Modi, Monica N., Sheallah Palmer, and Alicia Armstrong. 2014. "The Role of Violence against Women Act in Addressing Intimate Partner Violence: A Public Health Issue." *Journal of Women's Health* 23 (3): 253–259.

Moghe, Sonia, and Rosa Flores. December 13, 2018. "Shelters holding nearly 15,000 migrant children near capacity." CNN. https://www.cnn.com/2018/12/13/politics/migrant-children-us-custody/index.html.

Mogul, Joey L., Andrea J. Ritchie, and Kay Whitlock. 2011. *Queer (In)Justice: The Criminalization of LGBT People in the United States.* Vol. 5. Boston: Beacon Press.

Mor, Vincent, Jacqueline Zinn, Joseph Angelelli, Joan M. Teno, and Susan C. Miller. 2004. "Driven to Tiers: Socioeconomic and Racial Disparities in the Quality of Nursing Home Care." *Milbank Quarterly* 82 (2): 227–256.

Mulligan, Jessica. 2016. "Insurance Accounts: The Cultural Logics of Health Care Financing." *Medical Anthropology Quarterly* 30 (1): 37–61.

Nasdaq GlobalNewswire. 2016. "CCA Reports Fourth Quarter and Full Year 2015 Financial Results." February 10, 2016. http://www.globenewswire.com/news-release/2016/02/10/809594/0/en/CCA-Reports-Fourth-Quarter-and-Full-Year-2015-Financial-Results.html.

National Center for Health Statistics. 2017. "Hospital Utilization (in Non-federal Short-Stay Hospitals)." https://www.cdc.gov/nchs/fastats/hospital.htm.

National Day Laborer Organizing Network. 2017. "Legalization." https://ndlon.org/legalization/. Accessed January 24, 2019.

New York Times. 2009. "Stopping Dialysis at the End of Life." September 18, 2009. https://consults.blogs.nytimes.com/2009/09/18/end-of-life-care-and-dialysis/.

Ngai, Mae M. 2004. *Impossible Subjects.* Princeton, NJ: Princeton University Press.

Nguyen, V. K. 2008. "Antiretroviral Globalism, Biopolitics, and Therapeutic Citizenship." In *Global Assemblages: Technology, Politics, and Ethics as Anthropological Problems,* edited by Aihwa Ong and Stephen J. Collier, 124–144. Oxford: Blackwell Publishing.

Novak, Nicole L., Arline T. Geronimus, and Aresha M. Martinez-Cardoso. 2017. "Change in Birth Outcomes among Infants Born to Latina Mothers after a Major Immigration Raid." *International Journal of Epidemiology* 46 (3): 839–849.

Oberlander, Jonathan B., and Barbara Lyons. 2009. "Beyond Incrementalism? SCHIP and the Politics of Health Reform." *Health Affairs* 28 (3): w399–410.

O'Daniel, A. A. 2008. "Pushing Poverty to the Periphery: HIV-Positive African American Women's Health Needs, the Ryan White Care Act, and a Political Economy of Service Provision." *Transforming Anthropology* 16 (2): 112–127.

Odem, Mary. 2008. "Unsettled in the Suburbs: Latino Immigration and Ethnic Diversity in Metro Atlanta." In *Twenty-First Century Gateways: Immigrant Incorporation in Suburban America,* edited by Susan W. Hardwick, Audrey Singer, and Caroline B. Brettell, 105–136. Washington, DC: Brookings Institution Press.

Office of Management and Budget. 2009. *OMB Bulletin No. 10-02. Subject: Update of Statistical Area Definitions and Guidance on Their Uses.* Washington, DC: Office of Management and Budget.

Okie, Susan. 2007. "Immigrants and Health Care—at the Intersection of Two Broken Systems." *New England Journal of Medicine* 357 (6): 525–529.

Olsson, Tore C. 2014. "Latino Immigration." *New Georgia Encyclopedia.* http://www.georgiaencyclopedia.org/articles/history-archaeology/latino-immigration.

Ong, Aihwa. 1995. "Making the Biopolitical Subject: Cambodian Immigrants, Refugee Medicine and Cultural Citizenship in California." *Social Science & Medicine* 40 (9): 1243–1257.

———. 1996. "Cultural Citizenship as Subject-Making: Immigrants Negotiate Racial and Cultural Boundaries in the United States." *Current Anthropology* 37 (5): 737–762.

———. 2006. *Neoliberalism as Exception: Mutations in Citizenship and Sovereignty*. Durham, NC: Duke University Press.

Ortega, A. N., H. Fang, V. H. Perez, J. A. Rizzo, O. Carter-Pokras, S. P. Wallace, and L. Gelberg. 2007. "Health Care Access, Use of Services, and Experiences among Undocumented Mexicans and Other Latinos." *Archives of Internal Medicine* 167 (21): 2354–2360.

Pallares, Amalia. 2014. *Family Activism: Immigrant Struggles and the Politics of Noncitizenship*. New Brunswick, NJ: Rutgers University Press.

Paluska, Mike. 2011. Study: HB 87 could cost state $1 billion? CBS 45. http://www.cbs46.com/story/16048333/study-hb-87-could-cost-state-1-billion

Parson, Nia, Rebecca Escobar, Mariam Merced, and Anna Trautwein. 2016. "Health at the Intersections of Precarious Documentation Status and Gender-Based Partner Violence." *Violence against Women* 22 (1): 17–40.

Passel, Jeffrey S., D'vera Cohn, and Anna Gonzalez-Barrera. September 23, 2013. "Population Decline of Unauthorized Immigrants Stalls, May Have Reversed." http://www.pewhispanic.org/2013/09/23/population-decline-of-unauthorized-immigrants-stalls-may-have-reversed/.

Patel, Jugal K. 2016. "Trump Wants Big Changes to Legal Immigration, Too—How Big?" *New York Times*, October 18, 2016. https://www.nytimes.com/interactive/2016/10/18/us/politics/trump-legal-immigration.html.

Pérez-Peña, Richard. 2017. "Former Arizona Sheriff Joe Arpaio Is Convicted of Criminal Contempt." *New York Times*, July 31, 2017. https://www.nytimes.com/2017/07/31/us/sheriff-joe-arpaio-convicted-arizona.html?mcubz=3.

Petryna, A. 2004. "Biological Citizenship: The Science and Politics of Chernobyl-Exposed Populations." *Osiris* 19: 250–265.

Pew Hispanic Center. November 7, 2012. "Latino Voters in the 2012 Election." http://www.pewresearch.org/wp-content/uploads/sites/5/2012/11/2012_Latino_vote_exit_poll_analysis_final_11-09.pdf.

Phillips, Kristine. 2018. "What a Doctor Saw in a Texas Shelter for Migrant Children." *Washington Post*, June 16, 2018. https://www.washingtonpost.com/news/post-nation/wp/2018/06/16/america-is-better-than-this-what-a-doctor-saw-in-a-texas-shelter-for-migrant-children/?noredirect=on&utm_term=.8d4e2e03d5a5.

Pizzi, Richard. 2009. "Atlanta Hospital May Limit Access to Free Care." Healthcare Finance News. January 5, 2009. http://www.healthcarefinancenews.com/news/atlanta-hospital-may-limit-access-free-care.

Plichta, Stacey B. 2004. "Intimate Partner Violence and Physical Health Consequences Policy and Practice Implications." *Journal of Interpersonal Violence* 19 (11): 1296–1323.

Posner, Karen L., William M. Gild, and Edgar V. Winans. 1995. "Changes in Clinical Practice in Response to Reductions in Reimbursement: Physician Autonomy and Resistance to Bureaucratization." *Medical Anthropology Quarterly* 9 (4): 476–492.

Pourat, Nadereh, Steven P. Wallace, Max W. Hadler, and Ninez Ponce. 2014. "Assessing Health Care Services Used by California's Undocumented Immigrant Population in 2010." *Health Affairs* 33 (5): 840–847.

Powell, Benjamin. 2012. "The Law Of Unintended Consequences: Georgia's Immigration Law Backfires." *Forbes*. http://www.forbes.com/sites/realspin/2012/05/17/the-law-of-unintended-consequences-georgias-immigration-law-backfires/.

Project South. n.d. "History of Anti-immigrant Legislation in Georgia 2006–Present." Accessed July 23, 2018. http://www.legis.ga.gov/Legislation/20132014/144806.pdf.

Pulido, Laura. 2008. "FAQs: Frequently (Un)Asked Questions about Being a Scholar Activist." In *Engaging Contradictions Theory, Politics, and Methods of Activist Scholarship*, edited by Charles R. Hale, 341–365. Berkeley: University of California Press.

Quesada, James, Laurie Kain Hart, and Philippe Bourgois. 2011. "Structural Vulnerability and Health: Latino Migrant Laborers in the United States." *Medical Anthropology* 30 (4): 339–362.

Raj, Anita, Jay G. Silverman, Jennifer McCleary-Sills, and Rosalyn Liu. 2004. "Immigration Policies Increase South Asian Immigrant Women's Vulnerability to Intimate Partner Violence." *Journal of the American Medical Women's Association (1972)* 60 (1): 26–32.

Reblin, Maija, and Bert N. Uchino. 2008. "Social and Emotional Support and Its Implication for Health." *Current Opinion in Psychiatry* 21 (2): 201–205.

Redmon, Jeremy. 2012. "Nearly 600 Government Agencies Face Penalties under Immigration Law." *Atlanta Journal Constitution,* September 18, 2012. http://www.ajc.com/news/news /local-govt-politics/nearly-600-government-agencies-face-penalties-unde/nSDtD/.

———. 2014. "DeKalb Jail Won't Comply with ICE Detainers under Certain Conditions." *Atlanta Journal Constitution,* December 4, 2014. http://www.ajc.com/news/news/state -regional-govt-politics/dekalb-jail-wont-comply-with-ice-detainers-under-c/njLsS/.

Rhodes, Scott D., Lilli Mann, Florence M. Simán, Eunyoung Song, Jorge Alonzo, Mario Downs, Emma Lawlor, Omar Martinez, Christina J. Sun, and Mary Claire O'Brien. 2015. "The Impact of Local Immigration Enforcement Policies on the Health of Immigrant Hispanics/Latinos in the United States." *American Journal of Public Health* 105 (2): 329–337.

Rickford, Russell. 2016. "Black Lives Matter: Toward a Modern Practice of Mass Struggle." *New Labor Forum* 25: 34–42.

Robert W. Woodruff Foundation. 2014. "About the Foundation." http://woodruff.org.

Roberts, Dorothy E. 2007. "Constructing a Criminal Justice System Free of Racial Bias: An Abolitionist Framework." *Columbia Human Rights Law Review* 39: 261–266.

———. 2010. "Collateral Consequences, Genetic Surveillance and the New Biopolitics of Race." *Howard Law Journal* 54: 567–586.

Rodriguez, Rudolph A. 2010. "The Dilemma of Undocumented Immigrants with ESRD." *Dialysis & Transplantation* 39 (4): 141–143. https://doi.org/10.1002/dat.20437.

———. 2015. "Dialysis for Undocumented Immigrants in the United States." *Advances in Chronic Kidney Disease* 22 (1): 60–65. https://doi.org/10.1053/j.ackd.2014.07.003.

Rose, Joel. 2018. "Doctors Concerned about 'Irreparable Harm' to Separated Migrant Children." NPR, June 15, 2018. https://www.npr.org/2018/06/15/620254326/doctors-warn-about -dangers-of-child-separations.

Rose, Nikolas. 2007. *The Politics of Life Itself: Biomedicine, Power, and Subjectivity in the Twenty-First Century.* Princeton, NJ: Princeton University Press.

Rose, Nikolas, and Carlos Novas. 2008. "Biological Citizenship." In *Global Assemblages: Technology, Politics, and Ethics as Anthropological Problems,* edited by Aihwa Ong and Stephen J. Collier, 439–463. Oxford: Blackwell Publishing.

Rosenbaum, Sara J., Peter Shin, Emily Jones, and Jennifer Tolbert. 2010. "Community Health Centers: Opportunities and Challenges of Health Reform." https://www.nhchc.org/wp -content/uploads/2011/09/KaiserCHCsandhealthreformAug2010.pdf.

Rylko-Bauer, Barbara, and Paul Farmer. 2002. "Managed Care or Managed Inequality? A Call for Critiques of Market-Based Medicine." *Medical Anthropology Quarterly* 16 (4): 476–502.

Sack, Kevin. 2009a. "For Sick Illegal Immigrants, No Relief Back Home." *New York Times,* December 31, 2009. http://www.nytimes.com/2010/01/01/health/policy/01grady.html.

———. 2009b. "Hospital Falters as Refuge for Illegal Immigrants." *New York Times,* November 20, 2009. http://www.nytimes.com/2009/11/21/health/policy/21grady.html.

Sacks, Mike. 2012. "Arizona Immigration Law's Supreme Court Oral Argument Set for April." *Huffington Post Politics,* February 3, 2012. http://www.huffingtonpost.com/2012/02/03 /arizona-immigration-law-_n_1253502.html.

Sainsbury, Diane. 2006. "Immigrants' Social Rights in Comparative Perspective: Welfare Regimes, Forms in Immigration and Immigration Policy Regimes." *Journal of European Social Policy* 16 (3): 229–244.

Salcido, Olivia, and Madelaine Adelman. 2004. "'He Has Me Tied with the Blessed and Damned Papers': Undocumented-Immigrant Battered Women in Phoenix, Arizona." *Human Organization* 63 (2): 162–172.

Sanders, Michael. 2004. "Urban Odyssey: Theatre of the Oppressed and Talented Minority Youth." *Journal for the Education of the Gifted* 28 (2): 218–241.

Sanford, V., and A. Angel-Ajani. 2006. *Engaged Observer: Anthropology, Advocacy, and Activism*. New Brunswick, NJ: Rutgers University Press.

Sassen, Saskia. 2002. "Towards Post-National and Denationalized Citizenship." In *Handbook of Citizenship Studies*, edited by Engin F. Isin and Bryan S. Turner, 277–292. London: Sage.

Scheper-Hughes, Nancy. 2004. "Parts Unknown Undercover Ethnography of the Organs-Trafficking Underworld." *Ethnography* 5 (1): 29–73.

———. 2006. "Consuming Differences: Post-Human Ethics, Global (In)Justice, and the Transplant Trade in Organs." In *A Death Retold: Jesica Santillan, the Bungled Transplant, and Paradoxes of Medical Citizenship*, edited by J. Livingston, K. Wailoo, and P. Guarnaccia, 205–236. Chapel Hill: University of North Carolina Press.

Schneider, J. A. 1999. "And How Are We Supposed to Pay for Health Care? Views of the Poor and the Near Poor on Welfare Reform." *American Anthropologist* 101 (4): 761–782.

Serrano, Alfonso. 2012. "Why Undocumented Workers Are Good for the Economy." *Time*, June 14, 2012. http://business.time.com/2012/06/14/the-fiscal-fallout-of-state-immigration-laws/.

Shahshahani, Azadeh. 2009. "Terror and Isolation in Cobb: How Unchecked Police Power under 287 (g) Has Torn Families Apart and Threatened Public Safety." American Civil Liberties Union of Georgia. https://www.aclu.org/other/terror-and-isolation-cobb-how-unchecked-police-power-under-287g-has-torn-families-apart-and.

Shear, Michael D., and Maggie Haberman. 2017. "Trump Defends Initial Remarks on Charlottesville; Again Blames 'Both Sides.'" *New York Times*, August 15, 2017. https://www.nytimes.com/2017/08/15/us/politics/trump-press-conference-charlottesville.html?mcubz=3.

Sheikh, Irum. 2004. "Racializing, Criminalizing, and Silencing 9/11." In *Keeping Out the Other: A Critical Introduction to Immigration Enforcement Today*, edited by David C. Brotherton and Philip Kretsedemas, 81–107. New York: Columbia University Press.

Shih, Kevin. 2017. "Trump's Wrong—Immigrants Promote Economic Growth." *Business Insider*, February 26, 2017. http://www.businessinsider.com/trumps-wrong-immigrants-promote-economic-growth-2017-2.

Shin, Peter, Jessica Sharac, Carmen Alvarez, and Sara J. Rosenbaum. 2013. "Community Health Centers in an Era of Health Reform: An Overview and Key Challenges to Health Center Growth." https://www.kff.org/health-reform/issue-brief/community-health-centers-in-an-era-of-health-reform-overview/.

Shoichet, Catherine E., and Curt Merrill. 2017. "ICE Air: How US Deportation Flights Work." CNN, May 29, 2017. https://www.cnn.com/2017/05/26/us/ice-air-deportation-flights-explainer/index.html.

Shore, C., and S. Wright. 1997. *Policy: A New Field of Anthropology*. New York: Routledge.

Simmons, Andria. 2014. "Atlanta's Ticket Traps: Slow Down or Pay Up." *Atlanta Journal-Constitution*, October 18, 2014. https://www.myajc.com/news/transportation/atlanta-ticket-traps-slow-down-pay/6JZfycaeaKQ3jYJGRxtHII/.

Singer, Merrill. 1995. "Beyond the Ivory Tower: Critical Praxis in Medical Anthropology." *Medical Anthropology Quarterly* 9 (1): 80–106.

Smith, Jennifer M. 2010. "Screen, Stabilize, and Ship: EMTALA, US Hospitals, and Undocumented Immigrants (International Patient Dumping)." *Houston Journal of Health Law and Policy* 10: 309–358.

Sommers, Benjamin D. 2013. "Stuck between Health and Immigration Reform—Care for Undocumented Immigrants." *New England Journal of Medicine* 369 (7): 593–595.

Southern Poverty Law Center. 2018. "Georgia's Unchecked Immigration Enforcement Review Board." March 7, 2018. https://www.splcenter.org/hatewatch/2018/03/07/georgias -unchecked-immigration-enforcement-review-board.

Stein, Fernando. 2017. "AAP Statement on Protecting Immigrant Children." American Academy of Pediatrics, January 25, 2017. https://www.aap.org/en-us/about-the-aap/aap-press -room/Pages/AAPStatementonProtectingImmigrantChildren.aspx.

Stuesse, Angela, and Mathew Coleman. 2014. "Automobility, Immobility, Altermobility: Surviving and Resisting the Intensification of Immigrant Policing." *City & Society* 26 (1): 105–126.

Sutton, Joe. March 16, 2012. "Mississippi lawmakers pass controversial immigration bill." CNN .com. https://www.cnn.com/2012/03/16/us/mississippi-immigration-law/index.html.

Swift, James. 2011. "Voices: Cobb's D.A. King Applauds H.B. 87." Patch, May 16, 2011. https:// patch.com/georgia/kennesaw/voices-cobbs-da-king-applauds-hb-87.

Ticktin, Miriam. 2006. "Where Ethics and Politics Meet: The Violence of Humanitarianism in France." *American Ethnologist* 33 (1): 33–49.

Tjaden, Patricia, and Nancy Thoennes. 2000. *Extent, Nature, and Consequences of Intimate Partner Violence*. Washington, DC: U.S. Department of Justice, Office of Justice Programs, National Institute of Justice.

Trevizo, Perla. 2011. "Dalton Couple Fights to Regain Custody of Their Five Children." *Chattanooga Times Free Press*, November 27, 2011. http://www.timesfreepress.com/news/news /story/2011/nov/27/couple-fights-immigration-to-regain-custody/64863/.

———. 2012. "Immigration Must Be Fixed, Leaders Agree." *Chattanooga Times Free Press*, June 12, 2012. http://www.timesfreepress.com/news/news/story/2012/jun/12/0612-b1 -immigration-must-be-fixed-leaders-agree/80087/.

Uggen, Christopher, and Jeff Manza. 2002. "Democratic Contraction? Political Consequences of Felon Disenfranchisement in the United States." *American Sociological Review* 67 (6): 777–803.

United States Census Bureau. 2017. "QuickFacts. Doraville city, Georgia." https://www.census .gov/quickfacts/fact/table/doravillecitygeorgia/PST045217.

United States Census Bureau. 2017. "QuickFacts. Cartersville city, Georgia." https://www .census.gov/quickfacts/cartersvillecitygeorgia.

———. 2010. "Profile of General Population and Housing Characteristics: 2010. Geography: Georgia." United States Government. http://factfinder2.census.gov/rest/dnldController /deliver?_ts=362243114179.

United States Congress. 1996. Personal Responsibility and Work Opportunity Reconciliation Act of 1996, Pub. L. No. 104-193.

United States Department of Justice. 2014. "Government Intervenes in Lawsuit against Tenet Healthcare Corp. and Georgia Hospital Owned by Health Management Associates Inc. Alleging Payment of Kickbacks." February 19, 2014. http://www.justice.gov/opa/pr /government-intervenes-lawsuit-against-tenet-healthcare-corp-and-georgia-hospital -owned-health.

U.S. Citizenship and Immigration Services. 2018a. "Victims of Criminal Activity: U Nonimmigrant Status." https://www.uscis.gov/humanitarian/victims-human-trafficking-other -crimes/victims-criminal-activity-u-nonimmigrant-status/victims-criminal-activity-u -nonimmigrant-status.

U.S. Citizenship and Immigration Services. 2018b. "Green Card for a Victim of a Crime (U Non-immigrant)." https://www.uscis.gov/green-card/other-ways-get-green-card/green-card-victim-crime-u-nonimmigrant.

Vargas, Edward D., and Maureen A. Pirog. 2016. "Mixed-Status Families and WIC Uptake: The Effects of Risk of Deportation on Program Use." *Social Science Quarterly* 97 (3): 555–572.

Viladrich, A. 2012. "Beyond Welfare Reform: Reframing Undocumented Immigrants' Entitlement to Health Care in the United States, a Critical Review." *Social Science & Medicine* 74 (6): 822–829.

Villenas, S., and D. Deyhle. 1999. "Critical Race Theory and Ethnographies Challenging the Stereotypes: Latino Families, Schooling, Resilience and Resistance." *Curriculum Inquiry* 29 (4): 413–445.

Wacquant, Loïc. 2001. "The Penalisation of Poverty and the Rise of Neo-Liberalism." *European Journal on Criminal Policy and Research* 9 (4): 401–412.

Wailoo, K., J. Livingston, and P. J. Guarnaccia. 2006. *A Death Retold: Jesica Santillan, the Bungled Transplant, and Paradoxes of Medical Citizenship*. Chapel Hill: University of North Carolina Press.

Walcott, Susan M., and Arthur Murphy. 2006. "Latino Communities in Atlanta: Segmented Assimilation under Construction." In *Latinos in the New South: Transformation of Place*, edited by Heather A. Smith and Owen J. Furuseth, 153–166. New York: Ashgate.

Walker, Kyle E., and Helga Leitner. 2011. "The Variegated Landscape of Local Immigration Policies in the United States." *Urban Geography* 32 (2): 156–178.

Warmerdam, Elizabeth. 2016. "'Papers, Please' Law in Arizona to Be Clarified." Courthouse News Service. September 15, 2016. https://www.courthousenews.com/papers-please-law-in-arizona-to-be-clarified/.

Warner, David C. 2012. "Access to Health Services for Immigrants in the USA: From the Great Society to the 2010 Health Reform Act and After." *Ethnic and Racial Studies* 35 (1): 40–55.

Washington Post Staff. 2015. "Full Text: Donald Trump Announces a Presidential Bid." *Washington Post*, June 16, 2015. https://www.washingtonpost.com/news/post-politics/wp/2015/06/16/full-text-donald-trump-announces-a-presidential-bid/?utm_term=.eb97956ee49e.

Weaver, Christopher. 2014. "Justice Department to Join Suit against Tenet Healthcare, Health Management Associates." *Wall Street Journal*, February 19, 2014. http://www.wsj.com/articles/SB10001424052702303775504579393584121938484.

Wedel, J. R., C. Shore, G. Feldman, and S. Lathrop. 2005. "Toward an Anthropology of Public Policy." *Annals of the American Academy of Political and Social Science* 600 (1): 30–51.

Wernick, Laura J., Alex Kulick, and Michael R. Woodford. 2014. "How Theater within a Transformative Organizing Framework Cultivates Individual and Collective Empowerment among LGBTQQ Youth." *Journal of Community Psychology* 42 (7): 838–853.

Wessler, Seth Freed. 2011. "Georgia Immigrant Couple Fights to Regain Custody of Kids." Colorlines, November 30, 2011. http://colorlines.com/archives/2011/11/ovidio_and_domitina_mendezs_lost.html.

West, Carolyn M. 2002. "Lesbian Intimate Partner Violence: Prevalence and Dynamics." *Journal of Lesbian Studies* 6 (1): 121–127.

White, Kari, Valerie A. Yeager, Nir Menachemi, and Isabel C. Scarinci. 2014. "Impact of Alabama's Immigration Law on Access to Health Care among Latina Immigrants and Children: Implications for National Reform." *American Journal of Public Health* 104 (3): 397–405.

Wickert, David. 2016. How the Olympics helped lure Latinos to Atlanta. *Atlanta Journal Constitution*.

Willen, Sarah S. 2007a. "Exploring 'Illegal' and 'Irregular' Migrants' Lived Experiences of Law and State Power." *International Migration* 45 (3): 2–7.

————. 2007b. "Toward a Critical Phenomenology of 'Illegality': State Power, Criminalization, and Abjectivity among Undocumented Migrant Workers in Tel Aviv, Israel." *International Migration* 45 (3): 8–38.

————. 2011. "How Is Health-Related 'Deservingness' Reckoned? Perspectives from Unauthorized Im/Migrants in Tel Aviv." *Social Science & Medicine* 74 (6): 812–821.

————. 2012. "Migration, 'Illegality,' and Health: Mapping Embodied Vulnerability and Debating Health-Related Deservingness." *Social Science & Medicine* 74 (6): 805–811.

Williams, Misty. September 1, 2011a. "Dialysis Patients Lose Access to Treatments Discontinued." *Atlanta Journal-Constitution*, 2011.

————. September 9, 2011. "Grady, Dialysis Provider Set Deal 3-Year Deal." *Atlanta Journal-Constitution*. https://www.ajc.com/news/local/grady-dialysis-provider-strike-year-deal/bUPxvxWl6AtvGrIhu2ISjP/.

Wilson, Jill, and Audrey Singer. 2011. *Immigrants in 2010 Metropolitan America: A Decade of Change*. Washington, DC: Metropolitan Policy Program, Brookings Institution.

Wong, Jessica, and David Mellor. 2014. "Intimate Partner Violence and Women's Health and Wellbeing: Impacts, Risk Factors and Responses." *Contemporary Nurse* 46 (2): 170–179.

Woolhouse, Megan. 2004. "Hospital Stops Issuing Long-Used 'Grady Card.'" *Atlanta Business Chronicle*, January 26, 2004. http://www.bizjournals.com/atlanta/stories/2004/01/26/newscolumn5.html?page=all.

Wynn, Barbara, Theresa Coughlin, Serhiy Bondarenko, and Brian Bruen. 2002. "Analysis of the Joint Distribution of Disproportionate Share Hospital Payments." RAND and the Urban Institute. http://aspe.hhs.gov/health/reports/02/dsh/index.htm.

Wyss, K., D. Whiting, P. Kilima, D. G. McLarty, D. Mtasiwa, M. Tanner, and N. Lorenz. 1996. "Utilisation of Government and Private Health Services in Dar Es Salaam." *East African Medical Journal* 73 (6): 357–363.

Yarbrough, Robert A. 2010. "Becoming 'Hispanic' in the 'New South': Central American Immigrants' Racialization Experiences in Atlanta, GA, USA." *GeoJournal* 75 (3): 249–260.

Yoo, Grace J. 2008. "Immigrants and Welfare: Policy Constructions of Deservingness." *Journal of Immigrant & Refugee Studies* 6 (4): 490–507.

Young, Rick. 2011. *Frontline*. Season 30, episode 2, "Lost in Detention." Aired October 18, 2011, PBS Distribution.

Zavella, Patricia. 2012. "Why Are Immigrant Families Different Now?" *Policy Reports and Research Briefs*. Berkeley: University of California, Center for Latino Policy Research. http://Escholarship. Org/Uc/Item/77k1morm.

Zayas, Luis H., and Mollie H. Bradlee. 2014. "Exiling Children, Creating Orphans: When Immigration Policies Hurt Citizens." *Social Work* 59 (2): 167–175.

Zuckerman, Stephen, Timothy A. Waidmann, and Emily Lawton. 2011. "Undocumented Immigrants, Left Out of Health Reform, Likely to Continue to Grow as Share of the Uninsured." *Health Affairs* 30 (10): 1997–2004.

INDEX

Note: Page numbers in *italics* indicate illustrations.

ABOUT THE AUTHOR

NOLAN KLINE is assistant professor of anthropology and co-coordinator of the Global Health program at Rollins College in Winter Park, Florida. He earned a PhD in applied anthropology and a master of public health from the University of South Florida. He has published research on immigration enforcement and health, farmworker health, and LGBTQ+ Latinx activism following the Pulse shooting in Orlando, Florida. He has also worked in interdisciplinary research teams examining structural barriers to human papillomavirus (HPV) vaccination among children of migrant farmworkers, and explored how to improve HPV vaccination through interprofessional collaboration between oral health providers and medical providers. Because Kline is an applied medical anthropologist, his work intersects with public health, policy, and activism.